White Cell Manual

White Cell Manual
Edition 5

Alan Winkelstein, MD (deceased)
Professor of Medicine
Hematology/Bone Marrow Transplant Program
University of Pittsburgh School of Medicine
Montefiore University Hospital
Pittsburgh, Pennsylvania

Ronald A. Sacher, MB, BCh, DTM&H, FRCPC
Professor of Medicine and Pathology
Chair, Department of Laboratory Medicine
Georgetown University Medical Center
Washington, DC

Sandra S. Kaplan, MD
Professor of Pathology
University of Pittsburgh School of Medicine
Pittsburgh, Pennsylvania

George Roberts, MD
Department of Pathology
King Faisal Hospital
Riyadh, Saudi Arabia

 F. A. Davis Company • Philadelphia

F. A. Davis Company
1915 Arch Street
Philadelphia, PA 19103

Printed in the United States of America

Last digit indicates print number: 10 9 8 7 6 5 4 3 2 1

Acquisitions Editor: Robert W. Reinhardt
Developmental Editor: Bernice M. Wissler
Production Editor: Jessica Howie Martin
Cover Designer: Louis J. Forgione

As new scientific information becomes available through basic and clinical research, recommended treatments and drug therapies undergo changes. The authors and publisher have done everything possible to make this book accurate, up to date, and in accord with accepted standards at the time of publication. The authors, editors, and publisher are not responsible for errors or omissions or for consequences from application of the book, and make no warranty, expressed or implied, in regard to the contents of the book. Any practice described in this book should be applied by the reader in accordance with professional standards of care used in regard to the unique circumstances that may apply in each situation. The reader is advised always to check product information (package inserts) for changes and new information regarding dose and contraindications before administering any drug. Caution is especially urged when using new or infrequently ordered drugs.

Library of Congress Cataloging-in-Publication Data

White cell manual Winkelstein, Alan, 1935-1996
    Alan Winkelstein, Ronald A. Sacher, Sandra S. Kaplan, and George Roberts. -- Ed. 5
      p. cm.
    Rev. ed. of: White cell manual / Dane R. Boggs, Alan Winkelstein.
  Ed. 4. c1983.
    Includes bibliographical references and index.
    ISBN 0-8036-0305-3 (pbk.)
    1. Leukocytes.   2. Leukocyte disorders.
  I. Sacher, Ronald A., 1946-. II. Kaplan, Sandra S., 1934-. III. Roberts, George, 1940-.
  IV. Boggs, Dane R.. White cell manual.
    [DNLM: 1. Leukocytes.   WH 200 W582 1998]
  QP95.B59   1998
  612.1'12--dc21
  DNLM/DLC
  for Library of Congress   97-50157
                                               CIP

Preface to the Fifth Edition

Alan Winkelstein, the senior author of this fifth edition of the **White Cell Manual,** dedicated this edition to Dr. Dane R. Boggs, who had been Professor of Medicine and Chief of the Division of Hematology/Oncology, University of Pittsburgh School of Medicine. He was a hematologist who inspired and mentored medical students, hematology fellows, and colleagues for over 30 years. Within the course of this work, he conceived of the need for a readily usable written teaching aid, and so outlined the first edition of the **White Cell Manual** in 1967. Although this was only a mimeographed text, it became widely used by several schools as an introduction to the function and fate of various white cells.

For the third edition, Dr. Boggs asked Dr. Winkelstein to coauthor this manual, and in this way passed the authorship torch to him. The third edition was the first one that was published and widely circulated. Each of these two men manifested the characteristics of a natural teacher who could see issues clearly, break them down into their component parts, and then lucidly rebuild the relevant components in effective communication with their students. Each approached teaching with a dedicated selflessness, for the sheer joy of inducing the transformation from confusion to understanding in the eyes of their students. In 1984, after a fourth edition was published but before another could be prepared, Dr. Boggs died. The revival of the **White Cell Manual** was not addressed until Dr. Winkelstein picked up the torch under the impetus of the newly developed curriculum at the University of Pittsburgh School of Medicine. He carried this project on to virtual completion before he too died in December 1996. His dedication to this project and his tireless efforts in ensuring its completion were an inspiration.

The new curriculum emphasizes self-teaching, and this new edition should serve as a reference source and an introduction to the important host defense mechanism vital to the understanding of clinical medicine. The manual explores current concepts in the morphology and function of the leukocyte system, the sites of production, cell distribution, cell life span, the functions of the different types of leukocytes, and changes that occur in representative diseases of these cells. Because the manual is designed as an introduction to leukocyte physiology, it should not be considered a comprehensive discussion of all topics. The reader can find additional information in the major hematology textbooks or the selected readings listed at the end of this manual.

The authors gratefully acknowledge the help of many colleagues who contributed ideas and time to this manual. We wish especially to acknowledge Dr. Edward Ball, Dr. John Lister, Dr. Tim Carlos, Dr. Bruce Rabin, Dr. Sandra Rosen-Bronson, and Dr. Sallie Boggs. Special thanks are also due for the administrative assistance of Judith Steenson, Patricia Sites, and Maria Torralba. We also wish to express our thanks and gratitude to our spouses, including Alan's wife, Ann P. Winkelstein; Heather Sacher; Dr. Morton Kaplan; and Tunus Roberts, whose encouragement and assistance were vital in completing this project. We would appreciate receiving any comments and criticisms, especially from colleagues using this manual in hematology-related course work.

Ronald A. Sacher
Washington, D.C.

Sandra S. Kaplan
Pittsburgh, Pa.

George Roberts
Riyadh, Saudi Arabia

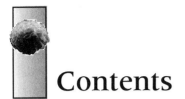

Contents

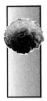

Chapter

1 Introduction

White blood cells or leukocytes are a diverse group of cells, found in the peripheral blood, whose major function is protection from environmental pathogens. These cells are broadly subdivided into two functional groups: those with responsibility for the ingestion and destruction of foreign particles **(phagocytes)** and those with responsibility for initiating specific immune responses against foreign antigens. Types of phagocytes include **neutrophils, monocytes, eosinophils,** and **basophils.** The various types of phagocytes have different functions and each behaves as a related but independent system. The immune effectors are **lymphocytes.** These cells are also subdivided into functionally specialized groups, each with a distinctive role in the immune defense system.

The functions of the phagocytic system are closely interrelated with those of the immune system. One of the most important interactions involves the processing and presentation of antigens by monocytes and dendritic cells (specialized antigen-presenting cells derived from monocytes) to immunologically competent lymphocytes. The stimulated lymphocytes then undergo a complex series of responses, which include:

1. The production of antibodies specific for the inciting antigen
2. The generation of cytotoxic lymphocytes capable of killing target cells expressing the inciting antigen
3. The release of soluble mediators capable of activating effector cells such as macrophages

Clinical Evaluation of Leukocytes

An evaluation of the leukocyte systems is essential in the management of all patients. Quantitative or qualitative alterations in the number of circulating leukocytes provide important information useful in the diagnosis and the management of a wide range of pathologic processes. Traditionally, medical laboratories report the

Table 1–1 • Normal Leukocyte Differential in Adults

	Percent	Total Number*
Neutrophils	45–74%	2.0–6.8
Band neutrophil	0–6%	0.1–0.8%
Lymphocytes†	22–50%	1.0–4.0%
Monocytes	0.7–7.5%	0.1–0.8%
Eosinophils	0–2%	0.0–0.2%
Basophils	0–2%	0.0–0.2%

*$10^6/\mu L$ or $10^9/L$ (calculated by multiplying the percent of the total white count/100).
†Includes T cells, B cells, and natural killer (NK) cells.

total leukocyte or white cell count (expressed as the number of white cells either per microliter or per liter) and a white cell differential, which lists the percentage of each type of white cell. For example, the total white count might be reported as 8000 cells/µL and the neutrophils as 63%. In practice, it is more valuable to consider the total number of cells of each type. In this instance, the absolute neutrophil count is 8000×0.63 or 5040 cells/ µL. The normal range for the concentrations of the various leukocytes in an adult is shown in Table 1–1.

Morphology of Leukocytes

Mature neutrophils (also called **polymorphonuclear leukocytes, PMN, polys, "segs"**) are the most numerous type of leukocyte in normal blood. Morphologically, they have a segmented nucleus with individual segments separated by a filamentous strand. On a Wright's stained smear (the usual cytochemical stain for evaluating white cell morphology), the nucleus appears dark blue with very heavily clumped chromatin. The abundant cytoplasm is slightly pink and contains "neutral"-stained (specific, secondary) and pink (azurophilic, primary) granules (lysosomes). The average number of segments is three, but a rare cell with as many as five segments can be found in normal blood.

    Band neutrophils ("bands"), slightly immature forms of neutrophils, are also present in normal blood. Except for their lack of filamentous segmentation, they are otherwise morphologically and functionally similar to mature neutrophils. In normal individuals, few band neutrophils are seen in the blood. An increase in their number is often the first indication of an acute infectious disease.

Lymphocytes, the second most numerous type of blood leukocytes, vary in size from slightly larger than red cells (erythrocytes) to larger than neutrophils. Almost all are small cells; the nuclear size of these small cells is often used as a reference for the size of normal red cells. A normal red cell has the same diameter as the nucleus of a small lymphocyte. Lymphocytes are usually round cells with a round nucleus, but both lymphocytes and erythrocytes may be oval or slightly indented and the nucleus may be deeply clefted. The cytoplasm is usually sky-blue but may be very light or very dark blue. The cytoplasm in small lymphocytes is often so scant that it is difficult to discern. In a small percentage of large lymphocytes, the cytoplasm is abundant and often stains deeply blue. Occasionally a few pink (azurophilic) granules can be discerned in the cytoplasm. Characteristically, the nuclear chromatin is heavily clumped, and nucleoli are discernible only in the larger cells. As discussed later, functional subtypes of lymphocytes cannot be distinguished by routine light microscopy; other procedures such as immunophenotyping (a technique designed to detect cell lineage by identifying specific membrane components) are required.

Monocytes may be among the more difficult cells to identify morphologically. They vary greatly in their size and overall appearance. The most reliable criterion for identification of a monocyte is the nuclear chromatin pattern. It is clumped, but the clumps are smaller in diameter and more elongated than in either a lymphocyte or a neutrophil. It appears as a lacy network. Monocytes are generally larger than neutrophils. The cell is typically round but may have irregular borders and evidence of pseudopods. Most often, the cytoplasm is blue-gray, but its color may be either bluish or neutral. It usually contains very tiny granules that are difficult to discern, but some monocytes are heavily granulated. Cytoplasmic vacuoles are often evident. The nucleus is classically described as kidney bean-shaped, but it may be round, oval, or highly indented. Monocytes may be confused with large lymphocytes or with immature neutrophils termed **metamyelocytes.**

Eosinophils and **basophils** are both present in the normal peripheral blood in very low numbers. Both are highly distinctive cells. They are approximately the same size as neutrophils. Eosinophils contain extremely prominent red (eosinophilic) granules; basophils have deep purple (basophilic) granules that often obscure the nucleus.

Immature myeloid precursors are normally present in the bone marrow but are not seen in the peripheral blood of normal individuals. They may, however, be present in the circulation in several pathological states. Neutrophil precursors are subdivided into different categories. In order of decreasing maturity, they are segmented neutrophils, band neutrophils, metamyelocytes, myelocytes, promyelocytes, and myeloblasts (Figure 1–1). Neutrophils, bands, and metamyelocytes are nondividing cells collectively designated as the **bone marrow maturation pool.** Metamyelocytes are cells slightly less mature than band neutrophils, with an oval or bean-shaped nucleus that lacks segmentation. These cells possess phagocytic properties and can be present in the circulation after extreme stresses such as severe infections. Metamyelocytes contain a full complement of cytoplasmic granules. They can be easily confused with monocytes.

The more immature myeloid precursors, the **myelocytes, promyelocytes,** and **myeloblasts,** are characterized by their ability to undergo mitotic division. Collectively, these cells are referred to as the **mitotic pool.** The actual distinctions among the various types of cells in the mitotic compartment should not be of major concern to students, but a general appreciation is important in understanding myelopoiesis. All cells in the mitotic pool have a round or oval nucleus. The nuclear chromatin is very fine in the myeloblast, slightly clumped in the promyelocyte, and more distinctly clumped in the myelocyte. Nucleoli are prominent in myeloblasts and promyelocytes, but less distinct in myelocytes. The cytoplasm is blue in myeloblasts and transforms into a more neutral color as the cell matures. Granules are absent in the myeloblast. Prominent azurophilic ("primary") granules are present in promyelocytes and "specific" or "secondary" granules appear at the myelocyte stage. These precursors tend to be larger than metamyelocytes.

The morphologic changes associated with myeloid maturation are depicted in Figure 1–2. These stages are somewhat arbitrary; cell maturation is a continuum and all processes may not occur at exactly the same rate. The development of granules is an orderly process; all primary granules are synthesized at the promyelocytic stage and all secondary granules at the myelocytic stage.

Plasma cells, the progeny of B lymphocytes, are cells that synthesize and secrete large quantities of antibodies. They are not

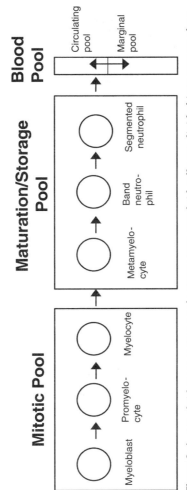

Figure 2–1. Myeloid maturation pools. Immature myeloid cells are divided into two pools: a mitotic pool, in which the cells have the capacity to divide, and a maturation pool, in which the cells no longer are able to proliferate but undergo a series of maturation steps leading to the formation of mature neutrophils. A storage pool, largely composed of bands and segmented neutrophils, serves as a reservoir from which cells can be released from the marrow to meet excessive demands, such as those occurring at times of severe infection.

5

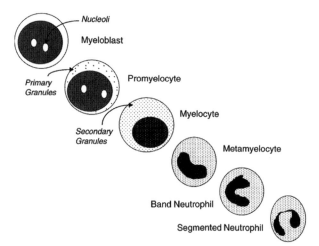

Figure 1–2. Morphological changes in myeloid cells during maturation. These changes can be summarized as follows: Immature cells (myeloblasts, top left) are large cells with a high nuclear/cytoplasm ratio. The nuclear chromatin is dispersed and prominent nucleoli are seen in the nucleus. The cytoplasm lacks distinctive granules and has a basophilic color. As the cell matures, the nuclear chromatin is condensed, the nucleoli are lost, the nuclear/cytoplasmic ratio decreases, and the cytoplasm gains features typical of a mature cell. Primary granules appear at the promyelocyte stage and secondary granules at the myelocyte stage. Only the myeloblast, promyelocyte, and myelocyte are capable of mitosis.

normally present in the peripheral blood but can be found in normal bone marrow and other organized collections of lymphoid tissues. They are round or oval cells with a rounded nucleus, located eccentrically in the cell. Cell size is quite variable; in general, the smaller the cell, the deeper the blue of the cytoplasm. There is usually a crescent-shaped, lighter-colored perinuclear clear zone. Nuclear chromatin is heavily clumped.

Identifying Subsets

Cell identification by light microscopic criteria has distinct limitations. To help define functional types of cells, several ancillary techniques are now commonly used. These include **histochemical stains,** which identify cytoplasmic or nuclear components unique to certain cell lines, and **immunophenotyping,** which detects the presence of cell membrane-associated components that distinguish specific cell types. For example, it has long been recognized that lymphocytes are morphologically homogeneous but functionally heterogeneous. Immunophenotyping can be used to group lymphocytes into three major subsets: **T (thymic-dependent) lymphocytes, B (bone marrow-derived) lymphocytes,** and **NK (natural killer) cells.** Furthermore, the T-cell subset can be further segregated into two functional groups, the **T helper/inducer cells** and the **T suppressor/cytotoxic cells.** Both immunophenotyping and histochemical procedures are important in distinguishing the cell of origin of an acute leukemia and other tumors of the lymphoid system.

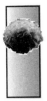

2 Stem Cells and Hematopoietic Growth Factors

Stem Cells

Hematopoietic cells, such as neutrophils, have finite life spans (Table 2–1). After their release from the marrow stores, neutrophils circulate in the blood for an average of 6 to 10 hours. Following this blood phase, they enter the tissues, where they may survive for an additional day or two. Mature neutrophils lack the capacity to proliferate, so the maintenance of a constant number of these cells depends on their continuous replacement with newly formed cells generated from precursor pools. The precursor cells arise from pools of primitive **stem cells** located within the bone marrow and other hematopoietic tissues.

Mitosis is the mechanism for new cell production. This proliferative process results in the formation of two daughter cells that are identical to the original cell. The capacity for **self-replication** is one of the defining characteristics of any stem cell system. The other necessary attribute in the hematopoietic system is that at least one of the daughter cells undergoes **differentiation,** leading to the formation of mature cells.

The stem cell compartment must be self-sustaining. In the steady state, for each cell that differentiates and thus leaves the compartment, another stem cell must be formed to maintain the pool size. This can be accomplished by one of two mechanisms (Figure 2–1). One involves **asynchronous cell division,** in which one daughter cell undergoes maturation while the other remains as a stem cell. In the other model, both daughter cells mature and the pool size is restored by the division, without maturation, of another stem cell. We do not know which process occurs, but

Table 2–1 • Features of Hematopoietic Cells*

- Mature hematopoietic cells have relatively brief life spans.
- Numbers are maintained by constant input of new cells from bone marrow.
- Life spans:

Neutrophils	6–10 hours (blood)
	1–2 days (tissues)
Monocytes	24 hours (blood)
	Few days (tissues)
Red cells	120 days (blood)
Platelets	7–10 days (blood)

- "One-way" circulation:
    - Egresses from marrow to enter blood
    - Egresses from blood into tissues or sites of destruction (e.g., spleen)
    - Unable to return to blood once removed from circulation

* These characteristics do not apply to lymphocytes.

in the steady state, the size of the stem cell pool remains constant.

The number of stem cells within the marrow is extremely small (less than 1% in the marrow and less than 0.1% in peripheral blood), and definitive morphologic identification of these cells is not possible. Most investigators believe that they resemble small lymphoid-like cells. The hematopoietic stem cells are contained within a population of hematopoietic cells that bear the CD34 antigen, which functions as a cell adhesion molecule. Although not all CD34$^+$ cells are stem cells, all stem cells are positive for this cell marker. Enumeration of CD34$^+$ cells has proven a valuable procedure for quantitating stem cell for marrow transplantation and peripheral blood transplantation.

Studies have established that stem and precursor cells are an extremely heterogeneous group. Some (**totipotent stem cells**) are able to form all the cellular elements of the blood, but others can mature only within distinct cell lineages. These various progenitors form a **cascade system** in which the most primitive stem cells feed into progressively more differentiated cell pools. The earliest stem cell, the totipotent stem cell, has the capacity of forming both lymphoid and hematopoietic cells. The lymphoid progenitors can differentiate into T, B, or NK cells, whereas those concerned

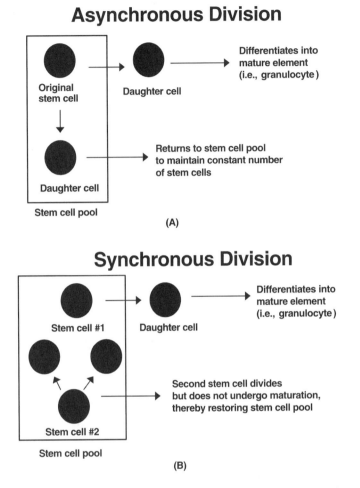

Figure 2–1. Two models by which the stem cell compartment can provide precursors for differentiated cells and yet remain constant in size. (A) In asynchronous stem cell division, one daughter cell matures while the second returns to the stem cell pool. (B) In synchronous cell division, after one stem cell has received a maturation signal, it leaves the stem cell compartment. A second stem cell then divides, giving rise to two new stem cells.

with hematopoiesis, **pluripotent stem cells,** give rise to phago-cytes, erythrocytes, and platelets (Figure 2–2). Totipotent and pluripotent stem cells are normally quiescent and become activated only when the more differentiated pools are depleted.

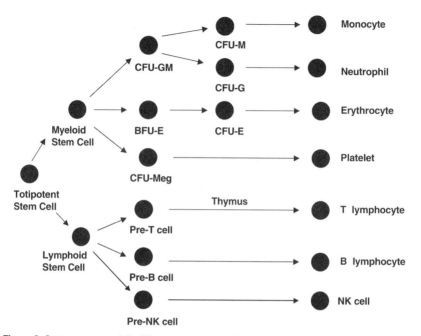

Figure 2–2. Current model of hematopoiesis. The earliest totipotent stem cell is capable of giving rise to both lymphoid and myeloid precursors. As the progenitors undergo progressive maturation, their capacity for differentiation becomes more restricted.

Progenitors are frequently recognized by their ability to form colonies in semisolid media; hence, they are often designated **colony-forming units (CFU).** Several different colony assays are used in both clinical and basic research to enumerate specific types of progenitors. The most widely used assays include those for granulocyte and granulocyte-monocyte colony-forming units (CFU-G and CFU-GM); for erythroid precursors (burst-forming units erythroid [BFU-E] and colony-forming units erythroid [CFU-E]); and for megakaryocytes (CFU-Meg). In addition, the activity of a cell closely related to the hematopoietic stem cell can be evaluated by a colony-forming technique for a colony-forming unit that produces granulocytes, erythrocytes, monocytes, and megakaryocytes (CFU-GEMM) or, in irradiated mice, spleen colony-forming units (CFU-S). Although several in vitro assays appear to measure even more primitive precursors, there are no universally accepted assays for the human pluripotent stem cell.

Cell Maturation

Kinetics of Cell Maturation

The kinetics of hematopoietic cell proliferation and maturation are complex. Several events occur in the processes of the differentiation of stem cells into recognizable precursors. These events include the proliferative expansion of precursors and their ultimate maturation into the differentiated effectors.

In the neutrophil system, for example, the CFU-G, a progenitor cell restricted to the neutrophil line, undergoes a series of divisions and maturation events ultimately leading to recognizable precursor myeloid cells. As discussed in Chapter 1, the earliest precursor, the myeloblast, differentiates into the promyelocyte, which in turn matures into the myelocyte. These early cells—the myeloblasts, promyelocytes, and myelocytes—collectively form the **proliferating pool** or **mitotic pool.** As the name implies, cells in this pool have the capacity to undergo mitotic division. The myeloblast has the most extensive capacity for repetitive cell division. With each division, the daughter cells become more restricted in their proliferative responses, and this restriction is accompanied by morphologic and functional evidence of maturation.

After completion of their proliferative expansion, the daughter cells enter the **maturation/storage pool.** Maturation within this compartment primarily involves the acquisition of the morphologic and functional features of mature neutrophils. This pool also serves as an important buffer. At times of increased demand for neutrophils (such as during an acute infection), cells from the storage pool can be released into the circulation. The more mature cells are released first. Except in instances of extreme demand, the cells that have just entered the storage pool are not released into the blood. In a normal person, the neutrophil reserves in the storage pool are huge. The storage pool contains 90% of the body's total neutrophils. Only 10% of the total neutrophil mass is present in the blood. The blood neutrophil pool consists of a **marginal pool,** in which cells are loosely and reversibly adherent to vessel walls, and a **circulating pool,** in which the cells are free in the circulation. The marginal and circulating pools are in equilibrium, and cells can move from one compartment to the other.

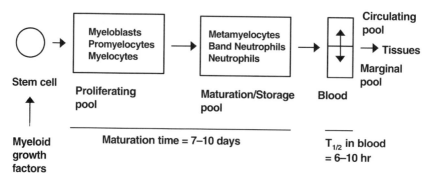

Figure 2–3. Kinetics of myeloid maturation.

Maturation of the cell from a myeloblast to a mature neutrophil requires 7 to 10 days (Figure 2–3). This time delay is essential in understanding the changes in blood neutrophils that occur in response to toxic injuries to the marrow. The classic example is seen in patients receiving cytotoxic chemotherapy for cancer. Drugs of this type are designed to selectively kill proliferating cells; thus, they act to destroy the mitotic pool. They do not injure cells that lack the capacity to divide; therefore they do not affect either cells in the storage pool or circulating neutrophils. Thus the storage pool serves as a buffer and neutropenia does not occur until cells in the storage pool mature and are released into the circulation. The presence of this storage pool accounts for the 7- to 10-day delay in the occurrence of neutropenia after cytotoxic therapy (Figure 2–4).

Recovery after a toxic injury first requires the reestablishment of the proliferating pool of cells. Once formed, these cells must multiply to restore the size of the pool and subsequently mature into cells that make up the storage pool. Only then are they released into the blood. Thus, the period of neutropenia after chemotherapy starts after a 7- to 10-day interval and persists for the same length of time.

Hematopoietic Growth Factors

Hematopoiesis is controlled by a series of soluble growth factors. More than 40 such factors have been identified and include both

Changes in Neutrophil Counts after Chemotherapy

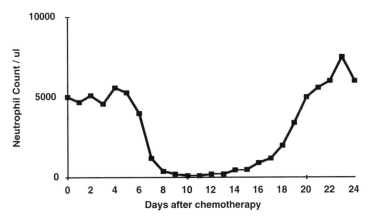

Figure 2–4. Sequential changes in neutrophil count in a patient receiving cytotoxic cancer chemotherapy drugs on day 0. Note that the nadir of the neutrophil count occurs approximately 10 days after drug administration and recovery is complete by day 21.

positive and negative regulators of hematopoiesis. Many of these factors have been cloned by recombinant DNA technology, so they can be produced in large quantities and used therapeutically. The principal indications for treatment with a recombinant growth factor are:

1. A deficiency of the factor, such as a lack of erythropoietin in chronic renal disease
2. An abnormal target cell that can respond to pharmacological but not physiological doses of an agent
3. To limit the duration of cytopenias following cancer chemotherapy

Currently, the most important factors regulating hematopoiesis are:

- Colony-stimulating factors (CSF)
  - Granulocyte (G-CSF)

- Granulocyte-macrophage (GM-CSF)
- Macrophage (M-CSF)
- Erythropoietin
- Thrombopoietin (TPO)
- Interleukin 3
- Stem cell factor (also called c-kit ligand, Steel factor, or mast cell growth factor)
- The interleukins, including IL-2, IL-6, IL-11, and IL-12

Certain general principles apply to most hematopoietic growth factors (Table 2–2). All are glycoproteins that are active at extremely low concentrations. Their ability to stimulate target cells depends on their binding to a small number of high-affinity receptors. Although their principal function is to stimulate proliferation and/or maturation of stem cells and progenitors, most hematopoietic growth factors possess multiple biological activities. They can promote the growth of different cell lineages and different stages of development within a single lineage. In some cases, they can also stimulate the growth of neoplastic counterparts of normal cells. For example, the primary function of GM-CSF is to induce the proliferation of myeloid stem cells and granulocyte/monocyte progenitors, but it can also promote the proliferation of both eosinophils and platelet precursors and can induce growth of some acute myeloblastic leukemic cells. The only factor that appears to have high-

---

Table 2–2 • General Properties of Hematopoietic Growth Factors

- Glycoproteins
- Active at extremely low concentrations
- Bind to small number of high-affinity receptors
- Multiple biological activities:
    - Able to stimulate or inhibit proliferation/differentiation of hematopoietic progenitors
    - May stimulate growth of other cell lineages and neoplastic counterparts of targeted stem cells
    - Enhance functions of mature cells
- Synergistic activities (growth factors may act in combination to yield results that are greater than the sum of their individual activities)
- May act directly on targeted progenitor or indirectly through an intermediate cell

ly restricted target-cell activity is erythropoietin, which acts almost exclusively on erythroid precursors. Thrombopoietin also appears to have relatively restricted physiologic activities.

Growth factors can also enhance functional activities of mature cells. GM-CSF increases the phagocytic properties of mature neutrophils and macrophages. Hematopoietic growth factors can also synergize with each other. That is, two factors that alone would have negligible effects on a particular target cell may act together to stimulate its growth. Factors may act either directly on a specific target cell or indirectly by inducing another cell to produce factors that have specificity for the target cell. IL-1 acts indirectly as a granulopoietin by inducing monocytes and macrophages to release GM-CSF.

In addition to these growth factors, which act primarily on hematopoietic precursors, there is a large and growing series of soluble mediators, the **interleukins.** These small proteins and glycoproteins are essential in all aspects of host defenses. They contribute to both hematopoiesis and lymphopoiesis, alter the activated states of monocytes and other phagocytic cells, regulate the type and magnitude of immune responses, induce the synthesis of various acute-phase reactants associated with inflammation, and are responsible for the systemic manifestations of inflammation (e.g., fever, anorexia, fatigue). More than 15 interleukins and a long list of related compounds have been isolated and cloned. Table 2–3 is an abbreviated list of interleukins and other important soluble mediators. Interleukins can act in an autocrine, paracrine, or endocrine fashion. Autocrine means that the product acts on the cell producing it (e.g., IL-2 is produced by activated T cells and stimulates its own proliferation). When acting in a paracrine fashion, the mediator acts on nearby cells; endocrine activity affects cells distal to the site of production. Interleukins may further be divided into those arising from lymphoid cells **(lymphokines)** and those from monocytes **(monokines).**

One of the important effects of hematopoietic growth factors is to inhibit the process of **apoptosis,** or programmed cell death. Apoptosis is a genetically controlled means of eliminating many types of cells. Morphologically, it is characterized by cell shrinkage and degradation of nuclear DNA. Most growth factors induce signals that prevent apoptosis; for example, GM-CSF, IL-5, and erythropoietin protect the viability of neutrophils, eosinophils, and

Table 2–3 • Interleukins

Interleukins	Cellular Source	Principal Activities
IL-1	Macrophages, other antigen-presenting cells, other somatic cells	Stimulation of T cells; B-cell proliferation and Ig production; acute phase responses; phagocytic activity; inflammation; hematopoiesis; release of GM-CSF, G-CSF
IL-2	Activated T cells, NK cells	T-cell proliferation, B-cell proliferation and Ig synthesis, NK-cell activation
IL-3	T lymphocytes, mast cells	Proliferation of hematopoietic precursors
IL-4	T lymphocytes	Proliferation of B cells, T cells, mast cells, fibroblasts; isotope switching to IgG and IgE in activated B cells; G-CSF and GM-CSF gene activation; inhibition of monokine production
IL-5	T cells, mast cells	Eosinophil growth and function
IL-6	Macrophages, endothelial cells, fibroblasts, T cells	Stimulation of hematopoietic precursors, T-lymphocyte proliferation, B-cell differentiation and Ig secretion, acute phase responses, plasma cell growth
IL-7	Thymic and marrow stromal cells	Proliferation of pre-B cells and pre-T cells
IL-8	Macrophages	Neutrophil chemotaxis and activation, T-cell chemotaxis, histamine and leukotriene release, angiogenesis

Table 2–3 (continued)

IL-9	T lymphocytes	Proliferation of fetal hemato-poietic precursors, erythro-poiesis in adults, T-cell proliferation
IL-10	T cells, activated B cells	Inhibition of cytokine produc-tion by Th1 cells; suppression of cellular immunity; inhibi-tion of mononuclear phagocy-tosis, class II antigen expression; promotion of B-cell proliferation
IL-11	Stromal cells	Activities similar to IL-6; enhances T- and B-cell prolif-eration, stimulates hemato-poiesis, acute phase reactive protein synthesis
IL-12	Macrophages, activated	Activation of Th1 cells, prolif-eration of cytotoxic T cells and NK cells, interferon γ produc-tion, suppresses Th2 function
IL-13	T cells	Activities similar to IL-4 (no effect on T cells)
IL-14	T cells	High-mw B-cell growth factor; may promote growth of some B-cell lymphomas
IL-15	T-cell tumors, other cells	Proliferation of activated T cells, NK cells; proliferation and Ig secretion by stimulated B cells

Abbreviations: G-CSF = granulocyte colony-stimulating factor; GM-CSF = granulocyte-macrophage colony-stimulating factor, IL = interleukin; mw = molecular weight; NK = natural killer.

erythroid colony-forming cells. These cells express receptors for their appropriate growth factor, but in the process of maturation these receptors decrease in number, thereby releasing the cells from the protective effects and permitting apoptosis to occur. The process is necessary to maintain appropriate numbers of cells. A failure to decrease the number of receptors for these growth factors can result in leukemic accumulations of cells, as discussed in the next chapter.

Chapter
3 Stem Cell Diseases

Aplastic Anemia

The term **aplastic anemia** is used to describe an uncommon clinical problem characterized by pancytopenia (a deficiency of all types of all peripheral blood cells) in the presence of a bone marrow markedly deficient in all precursors. Aplastic anemia is not a single disease but a syndrome that can result from multiple causes. It can occur as a congenital abnormality (Fanconi's anemia). More commonly, it is an acquired disorder. Acquired aplastic anemia has been further classified as primary (idiopathic) or secondary to a known cause. Some causes include idiosyncratic reactions to drugs (e.g., chloramphenicol or phenylbutazone), exposure to toxic chemicals such as benzene, or, rarely, viral illnesses, particularly hepatitis B. The vast majority of acquired cases are considered idiopathic, indicating that the cause is not known.

Pathophysiologically, aplastic anemia may be caused by a marked deficiency of stem cells, by an abnormality of the marrow stromal elements that prevents them from supporting the growth and maturation of hematopoietic cells, or by the presence of abnormal immune responses suppressing the formation or development of stem cells or their progeny.

Severe aplastic anemia is characterized by extremely low blood counts (neutrophils less than 500/µL and platelet counts less than 10,000/µL). It has an extraordinarily high mortality rate. Over 80% of affected patients die within 6 months if not treated, usually from infection or bleeding. Bone marrow transplantation is the treatment of choice for younger patients who have a suitable donor (to be discussed later). For older patients or those without a suitable donor, partial or complete remissions have been achieved with the use of immunosuppressants such as cyclosporine or antithymocyte

21

globulin (ATG). In most instances, hematopoietic growth factors are ineffective in reversing the pancytopenia. Patients with less severe forms of aplasia may survive for several years, but complete recovery is rare.

Aplastic anemia must be distinguished from the transient aplasia that occurs following cytotoxic cancer chemotherapy. One of the major side effects of many drugs used to treat cancer is lethal toxicity for hematopoietic stem cells. As a result, patients treated with these agents have a dose-dependent but reversible suppression of hematopoiesis. Thus, this form of aplasia is transient, and normal hematopoiesis is restored within a few weeks.

Leukemia

Leukemia is not a single disease, but rather a term that usually indicates the presence of neoplastic leukocytes in the peripheral blood. Conventionally, it has been subdivided into two general types, acute and chronic. The initial distinction between the two was based on survival. Patients with acute leukemia typically survived only a few weeks to months, whereas those with a chronic form were likely to live for several years. With improved treatment, however, survival alone is no longer an adequate criterion. Patients with acute leukemia frequently outlive those with the chronic form.

Pathophysiologically, the major distinction between the two forms of leukemia is related to the ability of the malignant cell to differentiate. An **acute leukemia** is a clonal disease in which the malignant cell is able to proliferate but is blocked from maturing beyond a very early developmental stage. Thus, there is a "maturation arrest," generally at the "blast stage" of development (Figure 3–1). Because the leukemic cells retain the capacity to proliferate, the neoplastic cells progressively accumulate, replacing normal hematopoietic tissues, and leukemic cells are released into the circulation.

The malignant cells in a **chronic leukemia** are also the progeny of a clone of primitive cells with unregulated growth and proliferation. They differ from acute leukemic cells in that they are capable of maturation. Thus, in **chronic myelogenous leukemia (CML)** the neoplastic stem cells can mature into neutrophils, without the arrested development that characterizes an acute leukemia.

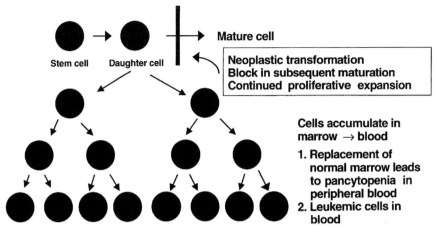

Figure 3–1. A maturation arrest as the basic pathologic process in an acute leukemia. The leukemic cells are able to divide, but daughter cells cannot undergo differentiation. As a result, "blasts" progressively accumulate in the bone marrow and are released or "spill out" into the blood. The increasing leukemic mass ultimately replaces the normal marrow elements, leading to anemia, neutropenia, and thrombocytopenia.

The distinctive feature of CML is a vast increase in all myeloid cells that leads to pronounced leukocytosis. Similarly, in **chronic lymphocytic leukemia (CLL)** there is a progressive accumulation of cells that morphologically resemble normal lymphocytes.

Acute Leukemia

Acute leukemias may also be distinguished by their cell lineage. Based on the origins of the neoplastic cell, acute leukemias are subdivided into **acute lymphoblastic leukemia (ALL)** and **acute myeloblastic leukemia (AML)**. This is the single most important clinical distinction. The two types of leukemia differ in their therapy, their response to treatment, and their prognosis. Both ALL and AML are further subdivided by morphologic, cytochemical, and immunologic features into defined subtypes. The most widely used classification system for acute leukemias is the French-American-British (FAB) system, which subdivides ALL into three categories and AML into eight (Table 3–1). In most circumstances, dividing acute leukemias into these subsets is more important in determining the comparability of different clinical trials than in the clinical management of individual leukemic patients.

Table 3–1 • FAB Classes of Acute Myelogenous Leukemia (AML)

Class	Characteristics
M0	AML without maturation or differentiation
M1	AML without maturation but with limited differentiation
M2	AML with partial maturation
M3	Acute promyelocytic leukemia
M4	Acute myelomonocytic leukemia
M5	Acute monocytic leukemia
M6	Erythroleukemia
M7	Acute megakaryocytic leukemia

Acute Lymphoblastic Leukemia

Acute lymphoblastic leukemia is the most common form of acute leukemia in children. The age peak is between 2 and 5 years, although older children and adults may also develop this malignancy. Based on the cell of origin, there are three different types of ALL: one in which the malignant cell has the characteristics of an immature T cell, a second in which it has features similar to those of an immature (pre-B) B cell, and a third in which the neoplastic cells resemble a cell arrested at the cytoplasmic immunoglobulin-positive (cIg^+) B-cell stage of development (Figure 3–2). The maturation of lymphocytes, the features associated with each developmental stage, and the concepts of an arrest at a particular developmental stage, resulting in each of the specific forms of ALL, are discussed in Chapter 5. A high percentage of both the B and T immature cells are positive for the intranuclear enzyme terminal deoxynucleotidyl transferase (TdT). This enzyme is involved in somatic generation of immunoglobulin and T-cell receptor diversity. TdT is not usually present in early myeloid cells or in AML.

The clinical manifestations of all forms of ALL result from the proliferative accumulation of lymphoblasts in the bone marrow, lymphoid tissues, and other anatomic sites. Because normal bone marrow hematopoietic cells are replaced by the leukemic elements, patients generally are anemic, thrombocytopenic, and neutropenic. The number of leukemic cells in the peripheral blood varies; in many patients it exceeds 50,000/µL. Because of the proliferative expansion of leukemic cells in the lymphoid organs, patients often show hepatomegaly, splenomegaly, and lymphadenopathy. Acute

Maturation Blocks in ALL

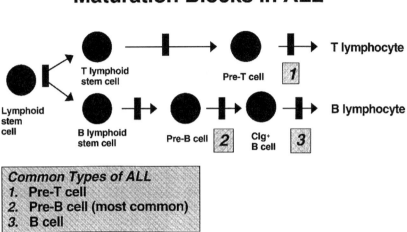

Figure 3–2. Arrests at different stages of lymphoid development, leading to the three major forms of acute lymphocytic leukemia (ALL).

lymphoblastic leukemic cells have a marked tendency to localize in extramedullary sites, particularly the central nervous system (CNS). This fact is important because systemically administered antileukemic therapy does not cross the blood-brain barrier and leukemic cells in the CNS are in a protected sanctuary.

ALL, particularly in children, is potentially curable. As explained in the next paragraph, with induction therapy followed by consolidation therapy and maintenance, as well as CNS prophylaxis, it is possible to induce remissions in up to 90% of affected children. Of these, more than 50% remain disease-free for prolonged intervals and are considered cured. Therapy for ALL in older children and adults is less effective, but with current multidrug regimens it is possible to obtain remissions in most patients. Nevertheless, recurrences are the rule, and only about 30% are cured.

Induction therapy refers to the initial treatment of leukemia and is designed to induce a **remission** (a condition in which leukemic cells cannot be identified by conventional morphologic techniques). **Consolidation therapy** consists of intensive courses of therapy aimed at eliminating any residual leukemic cells in a person already in complete remission. Either the same drugs used to induce a remission or a different regimen may be used.

Maintenance therapy is the prolonged administration of low doses of antileukemic therapy, designed to prevent any residual leukemic cells from replicating. **CNS prophylaxis** refers to treatment designed specifically to kill any leukemic cells that may have seeded (become localized) in the central nervous system.

Acute Myeloblastic Leukemia

AML is a group of clonal disorders caused by the malignant transformation and arrested development of an early myeloid precursor. The leukemic cells retain the capacity to proliferate; this leads to a progressive increase in tumor cell mass and replacement of the hematopoietic bone marrow by neoplastic cells. The incidence of AML increases progressively with age; it is the most common form of acute leukemia in adults. The peak incidence occurs in patients older than 65 years.

AML has been subdivided into primary and secondary forms, based on whether a recognizable predisposing factor can be identified. Such factors include radiation, exposure to toxic chemicals (such as benzene-containing compounds), or use of cytotoxic anticancer drugs. Another predisposing factor is the presence of a preexisting clonal hematologic disorder such as a myeloproliferative disease or myelodysplasia. In general, patients with secondary forms of AML are less likely than patients with primary AML to achieve remission with antileukemic therapy, and their survival rate is significantly lower. If patients with secondary AML do achieve remission, its duration is usually short.

Based on morphologic, immunologic, and cytochemical characteristics, AML (both primary and secondary) has been subdivided into eight FAB classes (see Table 3–1). Four of these classes (M0 through M3) indicate a block in normal myeloid maturation. The other four (M4 through M7) indicate a block in the differentiation of the neoplastic cells into hematopoietic lines other than neutrophils. The FAB classification system is useful in recognizing types of AML with unique features and determining the comparability of various investigational series. Nevertheless, the major clinical features and the general approach to therapy are similar for most patients with AML.

Acute promyelocytic leukemia (APL, M3) is a major exception with important clinical implications. This type of leukemia is characterized by a specific chromosomal translocation: a portion of chromosome 15 (containing the promyelocytic gene, pml) is translocated to a region of chromosome 17, to the gene that codes for the retinoic acid receptor, resulting in a maturation arrest at the promyelocyte stage. This translocation has important clinical implications. If the leukemic cells are exposed to a differentiating agent, all-*trans*-retinoic acid (ATRA), the maturation block can be circumvented, permitting the malignant cells to differentiate into neutrophils. This has led to a novel treatment for APL: patients can be induced to enter a remission with ATRA. This specific therapy represents the first instance in which treatment of a neoplastic disease is directed at inducing cell differentiation; all other cancers are treated with cytotoxic agents, surgery, or radiation therapy, aimed at killing or eliminating the malignant clone. Thus ATRA offers the promise of inducing a particular type of neoplastic cells to become responsive to the same factors that control the maturation and death of their normal counterparts. Unfortunately, the remissions induced in APL patients by ATRA are transient; without additional cytotoxic therapy the leukemia ultimately returns.

Clinically, patients with all forms of AML generally present with symptoms related to deficiencies in one or more of the normal cellular elements of the blood. Thus, cutaneous bleeding such as petechiae resulting from thrombocytopenia is a common manifestation. Likewise, undue susceptibility to infections or symptoms related to an anemia may be the initial manifestations of this type of leukemia. Affected patients may show enlarged livers and spleens caused by leukemic infiltrations, but such enlargement is observed less frequently in AML than in ALL. Not uncommonly, AML patients may also show cutaneous infiltration by leukemic cells. Unlike the situation in ALL, lymphadenopathy is rare in AML and CNS involvement tends to be a late manifestation.

The initial white blood cell count varies enormously from patient to patient. Some patients are leukopenic, with total white counts less than 1000/µL, whereas others have counts above 250,000/µL. Most, however, are in the range of 5000 to 30,000/µL. Ninety percent of patients with this disease have leukemic blasts in the peripheral blood, but in about 10% circulating leukemia cells cannot be identified. The bone marrow is always abnormal. In most cases it is markedly hypercellular because of the presence of a huge mass of leukemic cells. Concomitantly, there is generally a decrease in the number of normal hematopoietic precursors. To make a definitive diagnosis of AML, more than 30% of the marrow cells must be blasts.

Therapy for AML is less satisfactory than that for childhood ALL. Combined chemotherapeutic regimens can induce remissions in 50% to 70% of patients with primary AML, but recurrences are common. Even with intensive consolidation therapy, only about 25% of patients appear to be cured. Allogeneic or autologous bone marrow transplants (discussed later) may increase this cure rate.

The morphologic differentiation of AML from ALL is difficult. One morphologic feature that may help is the presence of **Auer rods** in the AML blasts. These are reddish, rod-shaped, cytoplasmic filaments that are believed to be aggregated lysosomes. Auer rods are present in only a subset of patients with AML and are particularly conspicuous in M3 AML. Both cytochemical and phenotypic characteristics of the leukemic cells can be used to distinguish AML from ALL. Table 3–2 lists some of the major characteristics that are useful for distinguishing the two types of leukemia.

Myelodysplasia

Myelodysplasia refers to another group of clonal disorders affecting hematopoietic stem cells. The primary characteristics of myelodysplastic syndrome (MDS) are a hyperplastic bone marrow, abnormalities in the maturation of precursors, and peripheral blood cytopenia. MDS has been called **preleukemia** because in many patients the disorder spontaneously transforms into acute myeloblastic leukemia. This transformation is unpredictable, however, so the term is inaccurate.

Pathophysiologically, the bone marrow in MDS is populated by a clone of defective stem cells. These cells undergo abortive maturation so that most die prematurely within the marrow. As a result, there are peripheral cytopenias and increased demands for hematopoietic cells, causing the marrow hypercellularity. The syndrome typically occurs in older persons and can be either primary (idiopathic) or secondary to exposure to the same agents associated with secondary AML.

MDS is subclassified into five FAB groups. Four reflect the number of blasts in the marrow: refractory anemia, refractory anemia with ringed sideroblasts, refractory anemia with excess blasts, and refractory anemia with excess blasts in transformation. The fifth subset is chronic myelomonocytic leukemia, a disorder characterized by a pronounced increase in monocytoid cells in the peripheral blood. Refractory anemia with ringed sideroblasts is a maturation abnormality with a classic morphologic appearance:

Table 3–2 • Features Useful in Distinguishing AML from ALL

Feature	AML	ALL
Morphology		
Cell size	Large	Small
Nuclear chromatin	Diffuse	Some clumping
Nucleoli	Multiple	One, often large
Cytoplasm	Moderate	Scanty
Auer rods	Sometimes present	Absent
Special Stains		
Esterases	+	−
Myeloperoxidase	+	−
PAS	− (except M6)	+
TdT	−	+
Immunophenotyping[*]		
CD33	+	−
CD13	+	−
CD14	+ (M4, M5)	−
CD7	−	+ (T cells)
CD5	−	+ (T cells)
CD2	−	+ (T cells)
CD19	−	+ (B, pre-B cells)
CD10	−	+ (pre-B cells)
Cytoplasmic μ	−	+ (pre-B cells)
Cytoplasmic CD3	−	+ (pre-T cells)
Cytoplasmic CD22	−	+ (pre-B cells)

ALL = acute lymphoblastic leukemia; AML = acute myeloblastic leukemia.
*Some leukemias do not run "true" to classic phenotype, but in addition:
    Some ALLs express CD33 or 13
    Some AMLs express CD7 (or 19)
    Some AMLs (up to 30%) express TdT.

erythroid precursors show a ring of iron granules surrounding the nucleus caused by the trapping of iron in mitochondria. In MDS, the greater the percentage of blasts in the marrow, the greater the likelihood that the disease will evolve into an acute leukemia.

Chronic Myelogenous Leukemia

CML is a clonal malignancy in which the principal manifestation is a persistent and often marked increase in the blood of both neutrophils and neutrophilic precursors. It is not unusual for the white count to exceed 100,000/μL. Unlike the situation in acute leukemia, in which the neoplastic cells are unable to mature beyond the blast stage, CML cells can fully differentiate. Therefore the differential count shows both mature neutrophils and myeloid cells at earlier stages of maturation. All stages of myeloid development, including occasional myeloblasts, are present in the blood. Many patients also have elevated platelet counts and may have increased numbers of blood eosinophils, basophils, and monocytes. In contrast, red cell production is typically suppressed, resulting in an aregenerative anemia. The bone marrow is extremely hypercellular because of a marked expansion in myeloid precursors. Extramedullary hemato-poiesis may be present and may result in enlargement of both the spleen and liver.

Pathophysiologically, CML results from an increased prolifer-ation of neoplastic hematopoietic stem cells that are not controlled by normal regulatory mechanisms. As a result, all myeloid cell compartments (mitotic pool, maturation/storage pool, and circulat-ing pools) are markedly expanded (Figure 3–3). In addition, imma-

Pathogenesis of CML

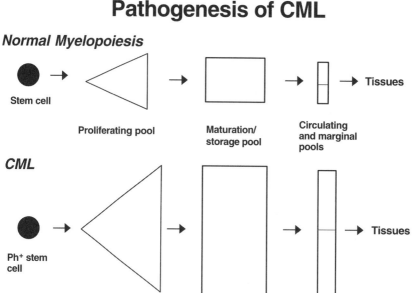

Figure 3–3. Comparison of the size of the mitotic, storage, and circulating pools for myeloid cells in normal subjects and in those with chronic myelogenous leukemia (CML). In CML, it appears that the major abnormality is a markedly diminished response of myeloid elements to normal regulators of hematopoiesis, resulting in an increase in all myeloid compartments. The myeloid precursors in CML are able to mature into neutrophils, in contrast to those in the acute leukemias.

ture cells, which are normally restricted to the marrow, are able to escape into the peripheral blood.

The hallmark of CML is the **Philadelphia (Ph) chromosome,** a translocation involving chromosomes 9 and 22. It is cytogenetically recognized by a shortening of the long arm of chromosome 22. Molecular genetic studies have shown that the Ph chromosome is a result of a translocation of the Abelson oncogene abl (c-abl) present on chromosome 9 to a region termed the breakpoint cluster region (bcr) on chromosome 22. As a result, a new gene termed the c-abl-bcr is formed; this codes for a high–molecular-weight tyrosine kinase, believed to be responsible for the abnormal cell proliferation. The Ph chromosome is present in approximately 90% of patients with CML. Most patients with Ph-negative CML have complex genetic rearrangements; by molecular genetic analysis, most also have the c-abl-bcr gene rearrangement.

Studies of patients with CML have provided valuable insights into hematopoiesis. Although the major clinical manifestation of the disease is the increased number of circulating myeloid stem cells, the Ph chromosome is also present in both erythroid and megakaryocyte precursors, and it may be found in certain lymphocytes. These findings suggest that it is caused by an acquired clonal abnormality affecting a pluripotential stem cell that is capable of giving rise to both hematopoietic and lymphoid cells. The Ph chromosome is not found in cells other than those involved in hematopoiesis; for example, it is not present in skin fibroblasts.

CML is clinically divided into three phases:

- A chronic phase, in which the major manifestation is a leukocytosis with orderly maturation
- An accelerated phase, characterized by increasing myeloid immaturity
- A preterminal blast crisis

The accelerated phase is often associated with other hematologic manifestations such as basophilia or thrombocytopenia. Patients may manifest systemic symptoms such as night sweats and weight loss. In the preterminal blast crisis, the disease is transformed into an acute leukemia. Although most of these acute leukemia transformations are myeloblastic, approximately one-third of cases are transformed into an acute lymphoblastic leukemia. This transformation further supports the concept that CML is a stem cell disease affecting the pluripotential stem cell.

The median survival for patients with CML from the time of diagnosis to death is 3 to 4 years. Newer treatments, including alpha-interferon, appear to prolong the chronic phase and therefore the life span. Bone marrow transplants are potentially curative.

Polycythemia Vera and Other Myeloproliferative Disorders

Polycythemia Vera

Polycythemia vera is also a clonal hematopoietic disorder characterized by dysregulated cell production. In this condition, the principal abnormality is the excess production of erythrocytes, but the disorder is a stem cell abnormality. Patients usually manifest concomitant increases in white blood cell and platelet counts. In vitro studies have shown that progenitor cells behave abnormally. Red cell colony formation occurs without the addition of exogenous erythropoietin. Normal erythroid precursors, in contrast, require this growth factor for colony growth.

Patients with polycythemia vera can survive for prolonged periods. Typically, most symptoms are related to poor tissue perfusion caused by an excessively high red cell mass, which results in increased blood viscosity and resistance to flow. Other clinical manifestations include plethora (a ruddy appearance) and splenomegaly. Polycythemia vera must be distinguished from other causes of increased red cell mass, including chronic hypoxia, erythropoietin-producing tumors (particularly renal tumors), and abnormal hemoglobins with a high affinity for oxygen. One of the distinguishing features of polycythemia vera is extremely low endogenous levels of erythropoietin. In contrast, secondary forms of erythrocytosis have either elevated or normal serum levels of this hormone.

Polycythemia vera can be managed by reducing the hematocrit with repeated phlebotomies, cytotoxic drugs capable of interfering with the proliferative expansion of erythroid precursors, or alpha-interferon. Patients appear to be at an increased risk of developing acute myeloblastic leukemia, a risk that is greatly heightened if they are treated with either alkylating agents or radiotherapy.

Essential Thrombocythemia

Another clonal myeloproliferative disease resulting from a stem cell abnormality is **essential thrombocythemia.** As the name implies, this disorder is primarily characterized by excessive production of platelets. There is often a concomitant leukocytosis and, in some patients, a mild erythrocytosis. Because of the increase in platelets, affected patients are at risk for either thrombosis or, paradoxically, bleeding. This bleeding appears to result from either defective platelet function or an inability to form a primary hemostatic plug because of their mass. Treatment is directed at reducing the abnormally elevated platelet count. This can be accomplished with cytotoxic drugs or interferon.

Agnogenic Myeloid Metaplasia

The third clonal myeloproliferative disease is **agnogenic myeloid metaplasia** or **idiopathic myelofibrosis.** This disorder involves excessive production of fibrous tissue in the marrow. The basic pathologic lesion is not known, but the abundant growth of fibrous tissue may be caused by the release of excessive amounts of a growth factor (such as platelet-derived growth factor) from an abnormal hematopoietic clone. Although the clinical features of myeloid metaplasia are diverse, patients generally develop marrow failure. Manifestations include massive splenomegaly, a bone marrow that cannot be aspirated because of the presence of excess fibrous tissue, and prominent extramedullary hematopoiesis.

Distinguishing among the Clonal Myeloproliferative Diseases

These three myeloproliferative diseases, together with CML, sometimes present a diagnostic dilemma. Patients often present with clinical or laboratory features that are consistent with more than one disorder. For example, prominent elevations in leukocyte counts and the presence of immature myeloid cells in the circulation may be found in any of the myeloproliferative diseases. Likewise, thrombocytosis and splenomegaly can be a major feature of all these disorders. All are associated with a variable predilection for transformation into acute leukemias. This transformation invariably occurs in CML.

CML can be distinguished by the presence of the Ph chromosome or the bcr-abl rearrangement. Characteristic cytogenetic abnormalities are not present in the other myeloproliferative disorders. One leukocyte intracellular enzyme, **leukocyte alkaline phosphatase (LAP),** also provides a valuable way of distinguishing CML from other myeloproliferative disorders or from a reactive leukocytosis (leukemoid reaction). The LAP score is almost always low in patients with CML, whereas patients with reactive leukocytosis, polycythemia vera, and essential thrombocythemia have elevated levels. Most patients with agnogenic myeloid metaplasia have either normal or elevated values for the enzyme. Table 3–3 compares the major features of the myeloproliferative diseases.

Table 3–3 • Major Features of Clonal Myeloproliferative Diseases

Feature	CML	Polycythemia Vera	Essential Thrombocythemia	Agnogenic Myeloid Metaplasia
Major clinical abnormality	Leukocytosis	Erythrocytosis	Thrombocytosis	Extramedullary hematopoiesis, marrow fibrosis
Typical age of onset	40–60	60+	40–70	60+
HCT	Usually ↓	↑	N or ↑	↓
WBC	↑↑↑	↑	↑	↓, N, or ↑
Platelets	N or ↑	↑	↑↑↑↑	↓, N, or ↑
Ph chromosome	+	–	–	–
LAP	↓	↑↑	↑	N or ↑
Tendency to transform into acute leukemia	++++	+	+/–	+

+ = positive; – = negative; ↓ = decrease; ↑ = increase, N = normal; CML = chronic myelogenous leukemia; HCT = hematocrit; LAP = leukocyte alkaline phosphatase; Ph = Philadelphia; WBC = white blood cells.

Bone Marrow Transplantation

Bone marrow transplantation is an important clinical modality for the treatment of several hematologic malignancies as well as non-hematologic, chemotherapy-sensitive malignancies and congenital and acquired disorders affecting the hematopoietic stem cell. In essence, transplantation involves the collection and preservation of normal hematopoietic stem cells to be administered after the patient's bone marrow, including its stem cell population, has been ablated by high-dose chemotherapy or irradiation. The transplanted stem cells may be obtained from either the same patient **(autologous transplant),** an HLA-matched donor **(allogeneic transplant),** or, if available, an identical twin **(syngeneic transplant).** After intravenous administration, the transplanted stem cells "home" (find their way) to the patient's bone marrow, proliferate, and ultimately reconstitute hematopoiesis.

This type of therapy is now widely used to treat aplastic anemia, acute leukemia, chronic myeloid leukemia, and certain forms of lymphoma, particularly those that recur after an initial course of potentially curative chemotherapy. Marrow transplantation is also used to treat selected inherited immune disorders such as severe combined immunodeficiency (discussed later), and has been used experimentally in patients with severe hemoglobinopathies such as sickle cell anemia and thalassemia.

More recently, marrow transplantation (or progenitor cells harvested from peripheral blood) has been extended to the treatment of metastatic nonhematologic cancers such as cancer of the breast. The treatment of these malignant diseases is predicated on the thesis that the tumor is susceptible to the lytic effects of cancer chemotherapy but that the toxicity of the drugs to the bone marrow precludes the administration of higher, curative doses. Marrow (or peripheral blood stem cell) transplantation can circumvent this problem by providing the patient with autologous stem cells that have not been exposed to lethal therapy by obtaining the stem cells before ablative treatment or by using allogeneic stem cells.

Autologous Transplantation

In an autologous transplant, the patient is the donor of the stem cells. This type of transplant is frequently used to treat patients with metastatic, chemotherapy-sensitive nonhematologic cancers (such as cancer of the breast); recurrent lymphomas; and acute leukemias that have achieved complete remission. The stem cells are collected from either the marrow or the peripheral blood. Collection from peripheral blood has been used with increasing frequency, particularly because progenitors can be readily mobilized into the blood by growth factors such as granulocyte colony-stimulating factor (G-CSF) or during the early recovery phase after cytotoxic chemotherapy. Peripheral blood stem-cell transplants have a distinct advantage over autologous bone-marrow transplants because hematopoiesis is reconstituted at a significantly faster rate and collection can be accomplished without general anesthesia.

The major limitation of autologous transplants is the possibility of infusing viable tumor cells admixed with the hematopoietic precursors. It is believed that tumor cells in numbers too small to be detected by routine cytologic examination may be sufficient to cause recurrence of the neoplasm. To try to circumvent this problem, many autologous marrow transplant protocols add procedures designed to eliminate residual tumor cells **("purging")** or to selectively transplant hematopoietic stem cells that have been separated from other marrow elements **(positive selection).** Purging has been accomplished with monoclonal antibodies that preferentially react with malignant cells (such as antibodies to CD15, an antigen expressed on many AML cells but not on normal early hematopoietic stem cells), or with chemotherapy agents that are active in vitro, such as derivatives of cyclophosphamide. Positive selection generally involves isolation of $CD34^+$ cells.

Allogeneic Transplantation

An allogeneic transplant involves the transplantation of stem cells from a normal donor. Allogeneic marrow transplantation differs significantly from transplantation of solid organs in that there must be HLA matching between the donor and the recipient. A solid-organ donation does not depend on such matching. As a result, most allogeneic transplants are performed using sibling donors. Statistically, a sibling has a 1:4 chance of inheriting the same HLA determinants from the parents as the prospective marrow recipient because the genes controlling HLA alleles are located on chromosome 6, and each sibling inherits one of the two chromosomes 6 from each parent (see Chapter 6). For individuals needing an allogeneic transplant but lacking a suitable sibling donor, national registries containing the HLA typing of huge prospective marrow donor populations have been established. Although the chance that any two randomly chosen individuals will be HLA-matched is extremely small, it is often possible to find an acceptable match with these large donor bases. The likelihood of successful matches has been further enhanced by the establishment of repositories of allogeneic cord/placental blood for transplantation. Placental blood has proven to be a rich source of hematopoietic precursors that can be readily harvested after detachment of the placenta

Allogeneic transplants pose a problem that is not encountered in autologous transplants, namely **graft-versus-host disease (GVHD).** This is a reaction caused by the presence of immunologically competent lymphocytes in the graft that are able to recognize and respond to the recipient's minor histocompatibility antigens. Because the recipient's immune system has been destroyed by the preparative chemotherapy, he or she is unable to eliminate these alloreactive cells. GVHD primarily affects the skin, liver, and gastrointestinal tract. Its major clinical manifestations include exfoliative dermatitis, liver dysfunction (sometimes leading to liver failure), and severe diarrhea. Severe GVHD has a high mortality rate, approaching 100%. The risk to the recipient can be significantly reduced by prophylactic immunosuppressive therapy (using drugs such as prednisone, cyclosporine, and methotrexate), but therapy for severe established GVHD is often not effective.

In addition to GVHD, there may be a beneficial immunologic reaction, termed **graft versus leukemia (GVL).** GVL was originally shown by comparing transplant results in various patients with acute leukemia. The recipient of a transplant from an identical twin (a syngeneic transplant, in which there is total histocompatibility matching) does not develop GVHD. However, recipients of such transplants show a significantly higher leukemic relapse rate than those who had an allogeneic transplant from a nonidentical sibling. These results suggest that, in an allogeneic transplant, there are immunologically competent lymphocytes that can destroy small numbers of residual tumor cells. This immunologic reaction may also be active against other types of malignant cells. Experimental efforts are in progress to define methods to augment the GVL reaction.

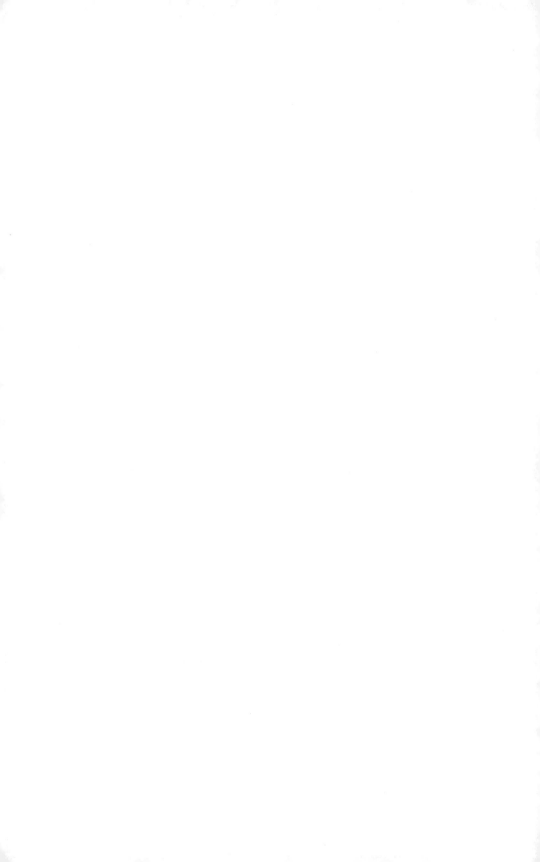

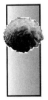

Chapter

4 Phagocytic Systems (Neutrophils, Monocytes, Eosinophils, and Basophils)

Localization, ingestion, and killing of invading microorganisms are the principal functions of the **phagocytic system.** This system also removes dead cells, debris, and noninfectious foreign particles. Localization of phagocytic cells to areas of inflammation or infection, the actual processes of ingesting particles, and the killing of microorganisms are complex functions. Neutrophils and monocytes appear to be the dominant cellular effectors of phagocytosis, but in specific types of infections, such as invasive parasitic diseases, and in allergic diseases, eosinophils may play a crucial role. Basophils are also considered a component of the phagocytic system, but their exact role is undefined. Because neutrophils and monocytes are essential to an intact host defense system, either a quantitative or qualitative deficiency in these cells means increased susceptibility to infection.

One of the basic processes that localize and destroy invading microorganisms is the formation of an inflammatory exudate. Through complex mechanisms involving the local release of soluble mediators of inflammation, metabolic activation, and granule effects (discussed in this chapter), neutrophils rapidly migrate to the involved area. This process occurs within hours after the initial injury. Once localized, these phagocytic cells can ingest and destroy the invading microorganisms. About 24 hours after the initial injury, however, the infiltrating neutrophils undergo degeneration and programmed cell death (apoptosis). They are subsequently replaced by monocytes, which can undergo further maturation into macrophages. Macrophages are even more effective phagocytes than monocytes. Concomitant with the migration of monocytes, an antigen-specific immune response is initiated as a result of infiltration by immunologically competent lymphocytes.

Neutrophils

Neutrophils are the most common type of cell in both the bone marrow and peripheral blood. They represent the first line of defense against invasion by pathogenic microorganisms. Their primary function is to localize and subsequently kill these organisms. As discussed later, a severe deficiency in the number of neutrophils markedly increases susceptibility to certain infections, particularly those caused by gram-negative bacteria, *Staphylococcus aureus,* and certain fungi, particularly *Candida* and *Aspergillus.*

The life cycle of neutrophils can best be appreciated by subdividing their production, maturation, and circulation into a series of contiguous compartments. As discussed previously, neutrophil precursors comprise the myeloid production and maturation/storage pools in the marrow. The **blood compartment** (Figure 4–1) can be considered a means by which these cells travel from the marrow

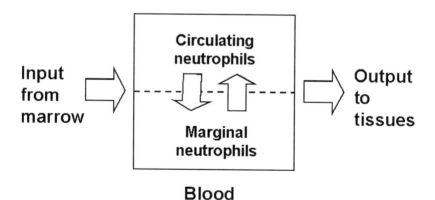

Blood

Figure 4–1. Neutrophils in the blood are present either free in the circulation (circulating pool) or loosely adherent to the vessel wall (marginal pool). The cells in these two pools are in equilibrium and can readily move from one compartment to another. In a normal steady state, approximately 50% of the blood neutrophils are in the marginal compartment. These cells are not enumerated in a blood count, so a normal person in a steady state has twice as many neutrophils in the blood as determined by the absolute neutrophil count.

to the tissues. This compartment is subdivided into a pool of circulating cells (the **circulating pool**) and a second pool that is loosely adherent to vascular endothelium (the **marginal pool**). Cells in this marginal pool can either return to the circulating pool or respond to peripheral mediators to leave the blood system and enter the tissues. In the tissues, neutrophils can be considered to be in an **extravascular pool.** Cells in this compartment cause local inflammatory reactions.

Neutrophil Kinetics

There is a dynamic equilibrium between blood neutrophils in the circulating and marginal pools. These cells move freely from one compartment to the other. In a normal person, about half of the blood neutrophils are in each compartment. Cells in the marginal pool are not static cells, irreversibly adherent to the vessel wall. They move freely over endothelial cells through the actions of various adhesion molecules (to be discussed later) and can either migrate into the tissues or return to the circulating pool. They migrate into the tissues by traversing between vascular endothelial cells.

The number of neutrophils recorded in a routine blood count reflects only the circulating compartment, not the neutrophils in the marginal pool. The blood neutrophil count can be altered by a shift of cells between the circulating and marginal pools, a shift that does not represent a true alteration in the total number of blood neutrophils. For example, if all of the neutrophils were to demarginate suddenly from the vessel walls, the neutrophil count would approximately double with no change in the total number of neutrophils in the blood. This is not an uncommon clinical situation. Epinephrine (adrenaline) is capable of causing rapid but reversible demargination, which accounts for the apparent neutrophilia seen in some acutely stressful situations. For example, a young child in an emergency room who is agitated and crying may have an elevated neutrophil count because of stress-induced demargination. If the count is repeated after the child becomes calm, the marginal pool has been restored and the neutrophil count returns to normal. Conversely, apparent neutropenia can be caused by an increase in the proportion of the blood neutrophils that are marginated (**pseudoneutropenia**).

Normally, the rate at which new cells enter the blood from the bone marrow is equal to the rate at which cells are being lost to the tissues. With radioisotope-labeled neutrophils, the disappearance

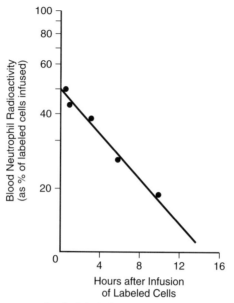

Figure 4–2. Disappearance of radiolabeled neutrophils from the peripheral blood over time, shown in a semilog plot. In these experiments, cells are removed, labeled with radioactive diisopropyl flurophosphate, and then infused into the same subject. These experiments indicate that neutrophils have a circulation time of 6 to 10 hours. Note that only 50% of the radioactive cells are in the circulation; the other 50% are in the marginal pool.

of injected cells can be followed over time. Figure 4–2 shows the disappearance of labeled cells. The curve is exponential, indicating that neutrophils are randomly disappearing from the circulation. A cell that has just entered the circulation from the marrow is as likely to leave as a cell that has been circulating for several hours. By contrast, red cell survival is not a random event; instead, these cells normally leave the circulation because they die of "old age." Kinetically, it has been determined that the average neutrophil spends 6 to 10 hours in the blood. Because of this brief intravascular life span, the total number of neutrophils in the blood is replaced by new cells from the bone marrow approximately 2.5 times each day (Figure 4–3). In comparison, red cells survive for approximately 120 days, so the erythrocyte mass is replaced every 120 days. After leaving the blood, neutrophils enter the tissues and appear to be capable of surviving for only a few days.

Neutrophils appear to have a one-way circulation. Once they enter the blood, they cannot return to the storage pool in the mar-

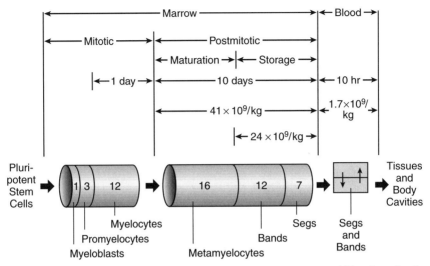

Figure 4–3. The kinetics and relative sizes of the bone marrow and blood pools of neutrophils and precursors in a normal person. The numbers on the cylinders indicate the cell ratios. Segs = segmented neurophils.

row. Likewise, after they leave the blood and enter tissues, they are unable to return to the circulation. Other phagocytic cells share this circulatory characteristic. By contrast, lymphocytes can both enter and leave the blood, so they are designated "recirculating cells." As previously discussed, mature neutrophils are "end-stage cells"; they are incapable of mitosis. Any increase in the total number of neutrophils must be met by an increased proliferation of cells within the myeloid proliferative pool.

Neutrophil Kinetics in Disease States
Three factors influence the blood neutrophil concentration:

1. The rate of neutrophil output from the bone marrow storage pool to the blood
2. The proportion of cells in the circulating pool as compared to the marginal pool
3. The rate at which cells exit from the blood into the tissues

The kinetics of neutrophils in infection (Figure 4–4) represent a balance between changing rates of outflow from the blood and inflow from the marrow to the blood. One of the earliest findings in specific infections, particularly those caused by endotoxin-secreting gram-negative organisms, is a transient neutropenia. This appears

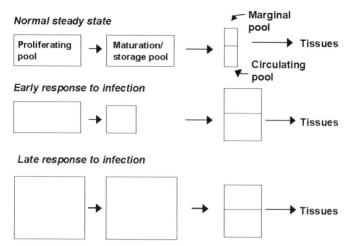

Figure 4–4. Neutrophil responses to infection: changes in kinetics and pool sizes.

to be caused by excessive margination. This form of neutropenia is usually transient. If it persists, it is a sign of a poor prognosis.

The typical finding in an infection is an increase in the number of neutrophils in the blood, a **neutrophilia.** The early increase in neutrophils results from a marked increase in the release of cells from the marrow storage compartment. The rate of movement of cells from the blood into the tissues also increases, but by less than the increase in the rate of release from marrow stores. As a result, the total neutrophil count rises. In addition, the number of circulating band neutrophils increases proportionately **(bandemia).** Thus the peripheral blood of a patient with an infection shows two characteristic changes: an increase in the total neutrophil count, and an increase in the ratio of band neutrophils to segmented neutrophils (Figure 4–5). As excess numbers of cells leave the storage pools, compensatory mechanisms designed to increase production are initiated. The release of endogenous hematopoietic growth factors such as G-CSF and GM-CSF increases. These induce the proliferation of myeloid progenitors and the subsequent expansion of the proliferating (mitotic) pool in the marrow. In chronic infections, a new steady state with expanded proliferating and maturation/storage pools is created (see Figure 4–4). It is not unusual to find that, in this new steady state, the ratio of band to segmented neutrophils returns to a normal range. By contrast, resolution of the infection is associated with a return to normal levels of the he-

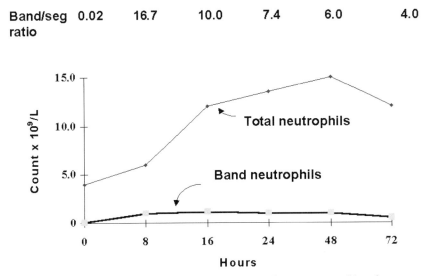

| Band/seg ratio | 0.02 | 16.7 | 10.0 | 7.4 | 6.0 | 4.0 |

Figure 4–5. Changes in absolute neutrophil count and percentage of band neutrophils in a patient with a typical acute bacterial infection. This changes the band/seg ratio as shown.

matopoietic growth factors and reestablishment of normal-sized proliferating and maturation/storage pools.

If the infection is severe, large numbers of neutrophils are present in the inflammatory exudates, leading to excessive demands for cells from the storage pool. This compartment may become exhausted, particularly in patients with preexisting marrow abnormalities and diminished marrow reserves. For example, alcoholic patients with folic acid deficiencies or patients undergoing cancer chemotherapy may have a markedly reduced marrow storage compartment. If they develop an infection, the excess demand for cells rapidly depletes this pool, leading to neutropenia. The concomitant reduction in the size of the proliferating pool limits its ability to replenish the storage pool, thereby prolonging and accentuating the neutropenia. With such a series of events, a relative deficiency in phagocytic cells arises at the site of infection. Thus it is not surprising that the development of neutropenia during the course of a severe, acute pyogenic infection, such as pneumococcal pneumonia, is a grave prognostic sign.

Neutrophilia
Besides infection, neutrophilia may result from other inflammatory stimuli or administration of certain drugs. Administration of

neutrophil growth factors G-CSF or GM-CSF induces a dose-related increase in the neutrophil count. These growth factors may also be used to mobilize hematopoietic progenitor cells for peripheral blood progenitor cell infusions.

Neutrophilia also occurs in patients with connective tissue diseases; other autoimmune disorders, myeloproliferative diseases such as polycythemia vera, myeloid metaplasia, and essential thrombocythemia; and often in association with malignancies. Pharmacologic doses of adrenal cortical steroids (corticosteroids) also induce neutrophilia. The mechanisms responsible for steroid-induced increases in neutrophils are complex. They include an increased release of cells from bone marrow stores and demargination of blood neutrophils from the marginal pool. Demargination tends to reduce the migration of these cells into inflammatory exudates, thereby decreasing the individual's ability to respond to pathogenic microorganisms. These effects of corticosteroids are transient. After a single intravenous dose of hydrocortisone, the peak neutrophilia occurs in approximately 4 to 6 hours and the counts generally return to baseline within 24 hours.

Neutropenia

Neutropenia, a reduction in the number of blood neutrophils, can result from several different mechanisms, including a shift of cells from the circulating to the marginal pool, an excess destruction or loss of preformed neutrophils, or a decrease in their production. A reduced rate of production is the most common pathologic basis. Decreased marrow synthetic activity can have many different causes, as shown in Table 4–1.

The severity of neutropenia is related to the risk of infection (Figure 4–6). There is relatively little increase in the risk of infection in patients with neutrophil counts greater than 1000/µL. As the neutrophil count progressively decreases, the risk for bacterial (particularly staphylococcal and gram-negative enteric bacterial) and fungal infections progressively increases. Most clinicians now use a level of less than 500 neutrophils/µL to identify patients at particularly high risk for infections. Clinically, a febrile illness in any patient with a neutrophil count below 500/µL must be considered a medical emergency. It is presumed that the patient is infected and the probability is high that the process will rapidly progress to septic shock and death. Broad-spectrum antibiotics must be started immediately.

Table 4–1 • Common Causes of Neutropenia

I. Decreased production
   A. Congenital
   B. Drug-induced
      1. Cytotoxic therapy
      2. Idiosyncratic
   C. Radiation
   D. Marrow replacement
      1. Neoplastic cells
      2. Fibrosis
   E. Deficiency of essential nutrients
      1. B_{12}
      2. Folate

II. Increased destruction
   A. Immune-mediated (antibody bound to neutrophil)
      1. Idiopathic
      2. Secondary
         a. Connective-tissue diseases (e.g., systemic lupus erythematosus, Felty's syndrome [rheumatoid arthritis, splenomegaly, and neutropenia])
         b. Lymphoproliferative neoplasms (e.g., chronic lymphocytic leukemia [CLL])
      3. Drug-induced (antibody against a drug bound to neutrophils)
      4. Neonatal (transplacental passage of antibodies)
      5. Cell-mediated neutropenia (suppression of myelopoiesis by direct cell contact, often mediated by T cells or NK cells)
   B. Severe infection (see text)

III. Pseudoneutropenia: shift from circulatory to marginal pool without changing total number of blood neutrophils (see text)

IV. Constitutional

Neutrophil Function

To successfully attack and destroy an invading microorganism, the neutrophil must leave the blood, migrate through the tissues to the site of infection, recognize the pathogenic organism, and then phagocytize, kill, and digest it. These events are conveniently subdivided into two broad categories, the migration cascade and the killing cascade.

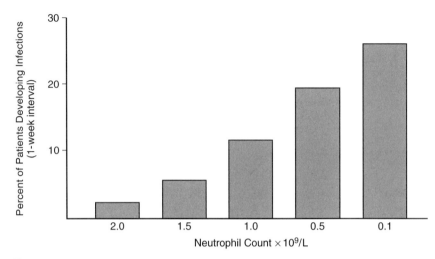

Figure 4–6. Risk of infection as a function of the total neutrophil count. Susceptibility increases markedly when the neutrophil count declines below 500/µL. (Adapted from Bodey, G.P., Buckley, M., Sathe, Y.S., et al (1966). Quantitative relationship between circulating leukocytes and infections in patients with acute leukemia. *Ann Intern Med,* 64, 328.)

The Migration Cascade

The migration of neutrophils from the blood into areas of inflammation is a process termed **recruitment.** This is a multifaceted process in which neutrophils initially attach to vascular endothelial cells and then migrate between these cells **(diapedesis)** through the basement membrane into the tissues and ultimately undergo directed migration to the site of inflammation.

Neutrophils emigrate from the blood into the tissues primarily through spaces between the endothelial cells lining the postcapillary venules. Although this is a continuous process, it has been arbitrarily separated into discrete phases (Figure 4–7). The first consists of slowing and a loose, reversible attachment of the circulating leukocytes to vascular endothelial cells. Because this is such a weak interaction, the flow of blood causes neutrophils to move or "roll" over the surface of the endothelial cells. Subsequent neutrophil-vascular endothelial interactions lead to firmer adherence to the endothelium. During this phase the neutrophil changes shape, converting itself from a spherical to a flattened form. Simultaneously, the cell becomes activated, as demonstrated by the expression of new membrane-associated proteins.

Next the neutrophil moves through the junction between adjacent endothelial cells. Finally it traverses the vascular basement

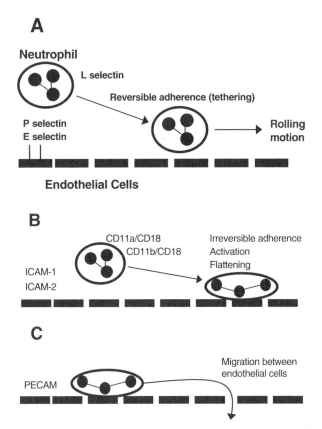

Figure 4–7. Stages of neutrophil adherence to vascular endothelial cells. (A) The initial phase consists of loose adherence (tethering), along with a rolling motion. This reversible phenomenon is mediated by the actions of the selectin molecules, L selectin on neutrophils and P and E selectins on endothelial cells. (B) The second phase consists of irreversible adherence, activation, and flattening of the neutrophils. These processes are primarily a result of the interactions of the integrin adhesion molecules on the neutrophil with the endothelial-cell CAM molecules. (C) The final phase consists of neutrophil migration between the junctions of adjacent endothelial cells. PECAM, another adhesion molecule, effects this process (see text).

membrane to migrate through the tissues to the site of injury. The passage of the cell through the basement membrane is a result of local digestion of the membrane, mediated partly by the release of intracellular enzymes such as proteases by the migrating neutrophil (discussed more fully on pages 54–60).

Adhesion Molecules. This process of neutrophil migration from the vascular system is mediated by a group of specialized ligands, termed **adhesion molecules,** and their receptors or ligands. Adhesion molecules are located on both neutrophils and endothelial cells, the latter indicating the vital role that the endothelium plays in cell migration. The initial rolling phase of adhesion (see Figure 4–7A) results from the interactions between the **selectin** family of cell adhesion molecules (CAMs) and their carbohydrate ligands. There are three types of selectins, called L, P, and E selectins. L selectins are expressed on neutrophils, whereas P and E selectins are located on endothelial cell membranes. P selectins are present in the Weibel-Palade bodies located in the cytoplasm of endothelial cells and platelets. On activation, endothelial components are rapidly translocated to the cell membrane. It appears that the initial adherence of neutrophils to endothelium is mediated primarily by the bindings of P and L selectins to their ligands, but these interactions are weak and readily reversible. It has been postulated that the third selectin, E selectin, may react with its carbohydrate ligand on neutrophils to produce a stronger, less reversible bond.

As just discussed, after selectin-mediated binding a series of interactions lead to the firm adhesion of neutrophils to endothelial cells, neutrophil activation, and alteration in their shape (see Figure 4–7B). These events depend on the binding of activated β_2 **integrins** present on neutrophils to their receptors, members of the immunoglobulin superfamily, the intercellular adhesion molecules (**ICAMs**) on endothelial cells. The neutrophil integrins consist of three heterodimer molecules, each possessing a specific alpha chain (CD11a, CD11b, and CD11c) and a common β chain (CD18). Thus, the three subtypes are designated CD11a/CD18, CD11b/CD18 and CD11c/CD18. It appears that the binding of CD11a/CD18 and CD11b/CD18b to their ligands on endothelial cells, ICAM-1, and perhaps ICAM-2, is primarily responsible for both the tight adhesion between neutrophils and endothelial cells and the shape changes in the phagocytic cell. The role of CD11c/CD18 on neutrophils has not been defined.

An important characteristic of the integrins is that during baseline conditions they are present in a less active form. Activation causes a conformational change in their structure. Conformational changes appear to result partly from the activities of several stimulatory molecules on the surface of endothelial cells. Another change that occurs during activation is the shedding of L selectin from neutrophils, which perhaps facilitates migration between endothelial cells.

Several inflammatory mediators that activate integrins on neutrophils have been identified. Two of the most important are platelet-activating factor (PAF) and IL-8. PAF is synthesized by endothelial cells within minutes after exposure to a variety of stimulatory agents and is subsequently expressed on the cell membrane. IL-8, a neutrophil chemotactic factor, is produced by stimulated monocytes and neutrophils; it appears to act after binding to the luminal surface of endothelial cells. Several other factors, including thrombin, histamine, and leukotriene-B_4, activate integrins.

The next process in neutrophil exudation is the migration of the neutrophils between adjacent endothelial cells. This process requires the activity of another adhesion molecule, platelet-endothelial cell adhesion molecule-1 (PECAM-1), another member of the immunoglobulin superfamily, although the exact mechanism by which it subserves this migratory function is not known. This adhesion molecule is located at the junction between endothelial cells.

One of the important clues to the significance of adhesion molecules comes from the study of two closely related disorders, termed **leukocyte adhesion deficiency (LAD) I** and **II**. Both disorders are characterized by profound defects in phagocyte emigration, chronic neutrophilia, and recurrent infections without the formation of inflammatory exudates. LAD I is caused by a deficiency of members of the CD11/CD18 family of adhesion molecules. LAD II results from deficiency of a selectin ligand.

Extravascular Migration of Neutrophils. Once the neutrophil enters the area of inflamed tissue, it may migrate back out (although it cannot return to the blood), die (and be phagocytosed by macrophages), or be immobilized while retaining functional activities. The integrity of the entire migration cascade can be tested in vivo by inducing a sterile inflammation and measuring the number of neutrophils entering the exudate. In humans this is usually assessed by the **skin window** technique. A small area of skin is superficially abraded and covered with a glass coverslip. Periodically, the coverslip is removed and stained and the attached cells are morphologically identified. Normally, within an hour a few neutrophils have migrated onto the coverslip. By 6 hours a fairly uniform monolayer of neutrophils has formed. By 24 hours, however, approximately 50% of the cells on the coverslip are monocytes. A modification of this technique allows quantitative measurement of neutrophil exudation. The abrasion is covered with a chamber filled with autologous serum and the total number of neutrophils migrating into the chamber is quantified. (More than 25×10^6 neutrophils normally enter a 1-mL chamber within 24 hours.) A reduced cellular response in a skin window, without neutropenia, suggests an abnormality at one or more stages in the migration cascade.

The overall integrity of the cascade can also be tested in vitro. One in vitro method involves the use of a specialized device, a **Boyden chamber**, which is a closed system with two sides separated by a porous filter. The holes in the filter are smaller than neutrophils, but sufficiently large (3 to 5 microns) to allow cells to deform and migrate from one side to the other. Neutrophils are isolated from the blood and placed in one side of the chamber. A chemotactic stimulus is then placed in the other side. During an incubation period, normal neutrophils are attracted toward the chemotactic stimulus and will be located either in the filter itself or on the side containing the stimulus.

Chemotaxins. **Chemotaxins** are naturally occurring or synthetic substances capable of inducing directed migration of cells. When a cell possessing a chemotactic receptor is exposed to a chemotactic gradient, it migrates in the direction of higher chemical concentration. During inflammatory reactions, naturally occurring chemotaxins are either released or generated. These include cleavage fragments generated by activation of complement, such as C5a and C5a-desarginine; secretory products of activated mast cells; cytokines and chemokines from lymphocytes, monocyte-macrophages, and the neutrophil itself; proteins generated from coagulation and kinin pathway activation; metabolites from lipo-oxygenation of arachidonic acid, such as leukotriene B_4; and products of invading bacteria and viruses. Synthetic chemotaxins are frequently used in experimental studies. The principal compounds are the formyl peptides such as formyl-methionyl-leucyl-phenylalanine, N-fMet-Leu-Phe (FMLP). FMLP is similar in structure to microbially derived chemotaxin and its activity simulates natural chemotaxins such as leukotriene B_4 and C5a.

The normal human neutrophil has approximately 50,000 receptors for FMLP. Binding of FMLP to its receptors initiates a complex series of poorly defined chemical events that result in a reorientation or polarization of cell shape from round to elongated/polarized. This change is associated with reorganization of cytoskeletal elements such as microfilaments and microtubules. **Polarized cells** have a broad, ruffled leading edge and a narrow tail (Figure 4–8). Another early change following binding of a

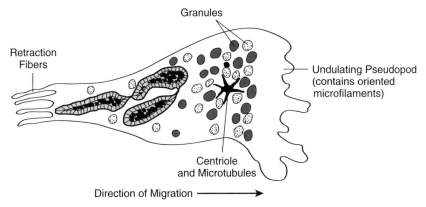

Figure 4–8. An "oriented" neutrophil. In response to a chemotactic stimulus, the neutrophil becomes oriented and moves toward the higher-concentration area of the chemotactic gradient. At the leading edge of the cell is an undulating pseudopod (termed a lamellaepodia), which is rich in actin- and myosin-containing microfilaments. Most granules are between the undulating pseudopod and the nucleus. The nucleus is at the rear of the cells, trailed by long "retraction fibers."

chemotaxin to a receptor on the neutrophil's plasma membrane is membrane ionic hyperpolarization, which occurs when ion flux (particularly calcium) accelerates. Other metabolic changes include alterations in synthesis and turnover of phospholipids (especially phosphatidylinositol and phosphatidylcholine), activation of phospholipases, and changes in cAMP and cGMP. Actin-myosin contractile proteins may mediate locomotion, and microtubules directed from the centriole orient and stabilize the cell contents.

Neutrophil movement has been characterized as "crawling" rather than "swimming." A surface is required for their locomotion. **Locomotion** is the form of random migration that occurs without orientation. The cells wander over a surface to which they are only loosely adherent. Orientation and locomotion can be separated by in vitro test systems. Low levels of magnesium in the suspending medium are required for locomotion, but not for orientation. When the chemotaxin is uniformly distributed in the medium suspending the neutrophil (i.e., when there is no gradient), orientation occurs but movement is random. However, movement in the presence of a chemotactic factor is more rapid and attachment is firmer than in its absence (**chemokinesis**).

The oriented neutrophil is very sensitive to chemotaxins. It moves directionally when presented with as small a gradient as 1% from head to tail. Its continued migration must involve repeated release from attached surfaces followed by rapid reattachment.

Continued recognition of a gradient may involve generation of new receptors at the leading edge of the cell and loss or inactivation of occupied receptors. As the neutrophil moves into an area of a higher chemoattractant concentration, it becomes less mobile. This loss of mobility is not well understood but probably results from the interaction of several factors. The chemotaxins themselves may be deactivated by a variety of products generated in the inflammatory response, including inhibitors released from neutrophil granules, and the higher concentration of chemoattractant induces the cell to produce oxidative free radicals such as superoxide (O_2^-) and peroxide (H_2O_2).

The Killing Cascade

The killing cascade is initiated when the neutrophil enters the vicinity of the foreign invader and ingests it. This is called **phagocytosis**, and is described more completely later. When the chemotaxin is a product of invading microorganisms, the neutrophil is attracted to the area containing the bacteria. Under this circumstance, phagocytosis of the bacteria can occur. Simultaneously with phagocytosis of the bacteria, the neutrophil granules merge with both the phagocytic vacuole and the cell membrane and granule contents are discharged into the vacuole (degranulation). The granules contain antibacterial substances and therefore participate in host defense in this manner, but because the granules are reservoirs of receptors for complement, formyl peptides, and other participants of the inflammatory reaction, the fusion of granules with the cell membrane also enhances the neutrophil's response to inflammatory mediators.

As with virtually all neutrophil functions, the events concerned with cell migration and killing are continuous and overlapping processes. For example, chemotactic stimulation has initiating effects on events concerned with the killing cascade, such as degranulation. By contrast, in the migration cascade some secondary granules fuse with the undulating pseudopod and are able to release their contents, such as collagenase, which may aid the cell in moving through tissues.

Self-regulation of the neutrophil's inflammatory response can occur at many points in the two cascades. That is, products formed or released by the neutrophil during its activation in inflammation can modulate the activation of other neutrophils. For example, the "killing complex" myeloperoxidase-H_2O_2-halide (to be discussed later) inactivates the chemotactic effect of C5a.

Phagocytosis. The process of killing generally begins with the internalization of the foreign particle. As already mentioned, this process is termed **phagocytosis** or **endocytosis**. Although the killing of microorganisms usually occurs almost simultaneously with phagocytosis, large organisms are sometimes killed without being phagocytized. For example, eosinophils are known to be able to kill parasites without actually internalizing them.

Before phagocytosis can occur, however, the process must begin with the recognition of the invader by the phagocyte and its attachment to the neutrophil cell membrane. These are closely linked events involving specific receptors. For example, if a bacterium has been coated by plasma proteins called **opsonins,** such as immunoglobulin (Ig) or the complement component C3b, it is attached to the neutrophil via receptors for the Fc region of Ig or for C3b. Attachment is followed by phagocytosis, lysosomal (granule) fusion, and degranulation.

The process of ingestion then proceeds with neutrophilic pseudopods protruding and surrounding the bacterium. This membrane movement is thought to entail the activities of microfilamentous actin and myosin, which also are responsible for the cell's crawling motion. When the leading edges of two pseudopods surrounding the bacterium touch, they fuse. By this fusion mechanism, the bacterium is internalized within a **phagosome** (Figure 4–9). The lining of the phagosome was initially the cytoplasmic membrane, but it becomes "outside in."

Oxidative burst (to be described later) and anaerobic granule-mediated killing mechanisms occur almost simultaneously. The granules of neutrophils are of three types: the primary (azurophilic) granule, secondary (specific) granule, and a poorly characterized tertiary granule, which contains gelatinase. In addition to chemical differences, the various types of granules also differ in their biologic activities.

Lysosomal (Granule) Fusion and Degranulation. In resting neutrophils, cytoplasmic granules are separated from one another and from the plasma membrane by a meshwork of actin-rich microfilaments. Simultaneously with phagocytosis, the filaments undergo focal lysis and the granules fuse with each other, with the cytoplasmic membrane in the area of bacterial attachment, and with the phagosome's membrane. The physical changes in these microfilaments occur because of chemical changes involving the

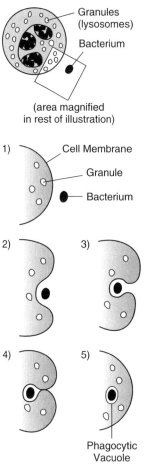

Figure 4–9. The physical process of phagocytosis.

membranes. As a result, the contents of the granules are expelled either extracellularly or directly into the phagosome.

All three types of granules are involved in the process of granule-phagosome fusion, but only specific granules are involved in **exocytosis**, in which their contents are released by fusion of the granule with the cytoplasmic membrane during the migration cascade. Certain enzyme contents, such as lysozyme, are contained in both primary and secondary granules, but myeloperoxidase and acid phosphatase are limited to primary granules. Alkaline phosphatase is localized to secondary granules. Granule contents not only participate in phagocytic killing, but also serve other purposes such as the digestion of previously killed organisms.

Respiratory Burst and Oxidative Killing. Coincident with phagocytosis, **respiratory burst** oxygen consumption accelerates markedly, generating cidal oxidants, which are derived from partial reduction of oxygen. Many substances activate the respiratory burst. Activation is energy-dependent and reversible but does not require either ingestion or degranulation. The initial step is the activation of a membrane-bound oxidase that has nicotinamide adenine dinucleotide phosphate (reduced) (NADPH) as its substrate (thus, NADPH oxidase). This oxidase catalyzes the reaction:

$$2O_2 + NADPH \xrightarrow{\text{(superoxide dismutase)}} 2O_2^- + NADP^+ + H^+$$

Hydrogen peroxide is, in turn, generated from the superoxide (O_2^-):

$$2O_2^- + 2H^+ \xrightarrow[\text{or via superoxide dismutase}]{\text{spontaneous}} H_2O_2 + O_2$$

NADPH is produced in neutrophils through activation of the **hexose monophosphate shunt (HMPS)**, which oxidizes glucose-6-phosphate to ribose-5-phosphate and CO_2 and, in the process, reduces NADP to NADPH. The H_2O_2 formed is needed for microbial killing in the phagocytic vacuole; any that diffuses into the cytoplasm is detoxified.

The detoxification of H_2O_2 also contributes to the HMPS by producing NADP:

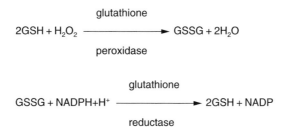

$$2GSH + H_2O_2 \xrightarrow[\text{peroxidase}]{\text{glutathione}} GSSG + 2H_2O$$

$$GSSG + NADPH + H^+ \xrightarrow[\text{reductase}]{\text{glutathione}} 2GSH + NADP$$

H_2O_2 can kill bacteria by itself, but its killing potency is greatly increased when it participates in another reaction catalyzed by the enzyme myeloperoxidase (MPO), derived from the neutrophil's azurophilic (primary) granules. In this reaction:

$$H_2O_2 + Cl^- + H^+ \xrightarrow{\text{myeloperoxidase}} HOCl + H_2O$$

In addition, H_2O_2 and O_2^- can interact to form another oxidizing radical, the hydroxyl radical (OH·). This is potentiated by the presence of iron. Superoxide itself is not a powerful killer, but its derivatives H_2O_2, HOCl, and OH· oxidize bacterial sulfhydryl groups and other membrane components and thus are potent bactericidal compounds. Chlorination of bacterial membrane components further contributes to bacterial death.

The killing capacity of neutrophils for bacteria, as studied in vitro, is considerable but not unlimited. More than 30 pseudomonas organisms can be ingested by a single neutrophil, but only about 20 are actually killed. As the ratio of bacteria to neutrophils is increased, the average number of bacteria killed per neutrophil increases, but the percentage of total bacteria killed is decreased. Thus, the more bacteria in an infection, the more neutrophils are required to clear them.

Anaerobic Killing Mechanisms. These mechanisms depend on small cationic proteins in neutrophil primary granules, called **defensins**. They kill bacteria by opening pores in bacterial cell walls. Other enzymes in granules that are capable of microbicidal action include lysozyme, arginase, and glucosidase in primary granules and lactoferrin in secondary granules. In addition, the microenvironment of the phagosome becomes acidic, and this pH change aids in the killing of specific organisms such as pneumococci. Not all pathogens are killed by the same biochemical mechanisms, which partially explains why specific defects may be associated with susceptibility to selected infections.

Digestion and Exocytosis. Finally, various granule constituents within the phagosome digest killed microorganisms, and the phagosome may be **exocytosed**, thus cleansing the cell of its debris. Actually, in the case of neutrophils, digestion and exocytosis may not be very important. Most neutrophils apparently die shortly after exudation, and are phagocytosed and digested by macrophages.

Pathologic Abnormalities In The Functional Cascades

Abnormalities of neutrophil function can be broadly divided into those caused by defects that are intrinsic in the neutrophil and those caused by external defects involving mediators of neutrophil function. Many congenital and acquired diseases (almost all of which are "new" diseases) are associated with each type.

Chronic granulomatous disease (CGD) is considered the prototype disease involving congenitally defective neutrophils. This relatively rare disorder was described as a clinical entity in the 1950s. It was then almost uniformly fatal in childhood, but now, with appropriate antibiotic treatment and the administration of interferon gamma, the length and quality of life have been dramatically improved. Affected children suffer from chronic granulomatous infections with bacteria ordinarily considered to be of low-grade pathogenicity, such as enterobacteriaceae, serratia, and coagulase-negative staphylococci. The patients have normal numbers of neutrophils, which appear to respond normally to infection. In 1966, however, Holmes and coworkers found that, although CGD neutrophils phagocytose bacteria, they fail to kill them. The defect results from defective function or absence of the NADPH oxidase that initiates the respiratory burst. As a result, H_2O_2 is not generated and is missing from the normal H_2O_2-halide–myeloperoxidase killing complex. Catalase-positive organisms are phagocytosed but not killed because catalase breaks down H_2O_2. Catalase-negative bacteria, such as pneumococci and β-hemolytic streptococci, produce H_2O_2 and thus engineer their own demise. The defect is not limited to neutrophils. Eosinophils and monocytes are also affected by the metabolic abnormality.

Initially, CGD appeared to be a sex-linked disorder that was seen only in boys. When the condition was observed in girls, other contributing factors were investigated. It was determined that NADPH oxidase (now called phagocytic oxidase or PHOX) actually consists of several components, all of which are required for activity but only one of which is inherited on the X chromosome. Genetically related defects in other components appear to account for the appearance of phenotypically similar diseases in girls.

Complement deficiencies can present as defects extrinsic to the phagocyte and are also associated with an increase in pyogenic infection. The prototype is a congenital absence of the opsonic component, C3. Lack of this component directly impairs phagocytosis and interferes with the generation of other components important for chemotaxis, such as C5a. Deficiencies of components of the classic pathway of activation leading to the generation of C3—C1r, C2, and C4—have been associated with abnormal neutrophil responses in vitro, but not with an increased susceptibility to infection. Presumably, this is because the alternate pathway of complement activation (Figure 4–10) is sufficient to generate C3, thus bypassing these classic pathway defects in vivo.

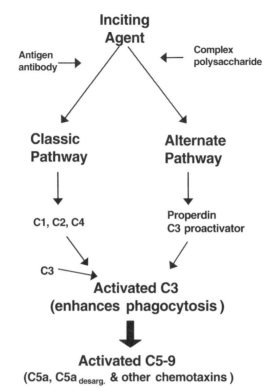

Figure 4–10. Mechanisms of activation of chemotactic components of complement.

Selected defects in neutrophil function are listed in Table 4–2. Some, such as CGD, routinely lead to death from infection without appropriate management. Others, such as acatalasemia or myeloperoxidase deficiency, are typically not associated with an increased susceptibility to infections. Absence of infection in the presence of a neutrophil defect presumably reflects the presence of alternative and overlapping pathways available to contain and kill invading organisms.

Diverse Effects of Neutrophils

Diverse consequences can result from inflammatory reactions and from the neutrophil's participation in them. The effect of neutrophil products on various tissues and constituents of tissues can be easily documented, but demonstration that they are a causative factor in human disease is more difficult. The following examples illustrate this.

Table 4–2 • Selected Defects in Neutrophil Function

I. Defects in migration cascade
   A. Congenital complement deficiencies
   B. Decreased generation of chemotactic factors
      1. Congenital
      2. Uremia
   C. Acquired production of chemotactic inhibitors
      1. Cancer
      2. Renal dialysis
      3. Chronic infections
      4. Idiopathic (IgG deficiency)
   D. Congential absence of a membrane glycoprotein
   E. "Job's syndrome": defective chemotactic response with "boils," increased IgE, eosinophilia, eczema
   F. "Lazy leukocyte" syndrome: undefined neutrophil defect, resulting in reduced release from the marrow associated with reduced adhesion and migration

II. Defects in killing cascade
   A. Chronic granulomatous disease
   B. Glucose-6-phosphate dehydrogenase (G6PD) deficiency
   C. Myeloperoxidase deficiency (increased susceptibility to Candida infections)
   D. Deficiency of H_2O_2 detoxifying enzymes

III. Defects with significant influence on both cascades
   A. Congenital absence of specific granules
   B. Congenital absence of actin polymerization
   C. Defects in microtubule assembly
   D. Diabetes and other causes of hyperosmolality
   E. Alcohol intoxication

IV. Defects in adhesion molecules
   A. Leukocyte adhesion deficiency, Type I (deficiency of Cd11/CD18 integrin)
   B. Leukocyte adhesion deficiency, Type II (deficiency of ligand for selectin)

Evidence is strong that the neutrophil plays a major role in the pathogenesis of the actual **gouty attack**. Gout is precipitated by uric acid, typically in the joint spaces. It usually occurs in individuals with elevated serum levels. The presence of uric acid crystals in the fluid attracts neutrophils and results in a sterile inflammation. Concomitantly, the exudate acidifies the joint fluid, resulting in more crystal precipitation and more inflammation. Thus, a vicious cycle is established. Colchicine in adequate doses will abort an acute attack of gout because it paralyzes neutrophils by poisoning their microtubules.

Another example in which neutrophils have an adverse effect on tissues occurs in hemodialysis. A highly predictable sequence of events occurs. The initial contact of the patient's plasma with the cellophane membrane of the dialysis apparatus results in complement activation. The $C5a_{desarginine}$ fragment induces aggregation of neutrophils in the blood. These aggregates become trapped in the capillaries or the precapillary vessels of the lungs. One consequence is an acute neutropenia seen shortly after commencing the dialysis procedure. This neutropenia is transient. It is rapidly reversed as neutrophil release from marrow stores is stimulated.

The trapped aggregates, however, can interfere with the pulmonary microcirculation. In patients with underlying lung disease, transient hypoxemia may result. Further, $C5a_{desarginine}$ promotes neutrophil adhesion as well as aggregation. This induces the release of neutral proteases from secondary granules. These proteases, in turn, can degrade elastin, collagen, proteoglycans, and basement membrane. The potential damaging effects of these enzymes can be modulated by local pulmonary antiproteases (which are inactivated by cigarette smoke). Because metabolic activities of the aggregated, adherent neutrophils are activated, potentially damaging superoxide, hydrogen peroxide, and hydroxyl radicals may also be released. Again, these may be inactivated before or during their release from the cell. Within a few minutes the neutrophil becomes "downregulated" and is refractory to $C5a_{desarginine}$, and deaggregation occurs.

Monocytes and Macrophages

Monocytes

Monocytes can be considered "immature" cells. They are produced in the marrow and released into the blood, and are destined to migrate into the tissues. Blood monocytes are 10 to 15 µm in diameter. Although they are phagocytes and ingest and kill bacteria, they are less effective than neutrophils. When they leave the bloodstream and enter tissues, they undergo terminal differentiation into more effective phagocytic cells called **macrophages**, including mobile and fixed-tissue macrophages. **Mobile macrophages** migrate through tissues to sites of inflammation. In contrast, **fixed-tissue macrophages** localize to the blood vessels; in certain specialized organs, they are assigned specific names, such as the Kupffer cells in the liver. Fixed-tissue macrophages are primarily responsible for removing microorganisms and debris, including dead cells, from the circulation.

Monocytes and neutrophils are both derived from a common stem cell and precursor, the granulocyte-macrophage colony-forming unit (GM-CFU). As shown in Figure 2–2, these cells subsequently mature into separate lineage-committed progenitors, one for neutrophils (G-CFU) and the other for monocyte/macrophages (M-CFU). On a Wright-stained bone marrow aspirate, it is not possible to distinguish the early monocyte precursors from myeloblasts. Early cells of both series have identical appearances, but the pool of monocytic precursors in the marrow is relatively small compared to the early neutrophils. Some distinction between precursors of neutrophils and monocytes can be made on the basis of staining for esterase (monocyctes are positive for nonspecific esterase) and by immunophenotyping. Early monocytic cells can be identified by the presence of CD14 antigen and HLA-DR expression. Monocytes also exhibit less myeloperoxidase.

Unlike neutrophils, monocytes do not have an appreciable marrow storage pool. The transit time of monocytes in the marrow is 1 to 3 days, and their time in the blood is slightly greater than that of neutrophils, averaging about 14 hours (range 8 to 72 hours). Like neutrophils, they randomly enter the tissues; their egress from the blood is independent of the time of entry from the bone marrow. Circulating monocytes, like neutrophils, appear to have a one-way circulation. Once they enter the tissues, they are unable to return to the blood. In contrast to neutrophils, monocytes in the tissues may have a prolonged survival, sometimes more than 80 days. In response to certain stimuli, these cells can undergo proliferative expansion; therefore they are not "end-stage" cells. The initial migration of monocytes from the blood to inflammatory exudates is slower than the migration of neutrophils, but ultimately monocytes become the predominant cell type, particularly as the inflammatory process is resolving. If the inciting stimulus is not removed, monocytes may aggregate to form giant cells and remain at the local site indefinitely. A local collection of aggregated macrophages is called a **granuloma**.

Monocyte production is controlled by numerous factors. Active inflammation is a potent stimulus to the generation of new monocytes. Within 12 hours their production can be increased fourfold. In addition, inflammation reduces the circulatory time to as little as 30 minutes. Monocytes can function in an autocrine fashion. They are able to elaborate growth factors such as GM-CSF and M-CSF, which, in turn, can promote their own proliferation.

Macrophages

Macrophages are much larger than monocytes—15 to 80 μm—and exhibit greater complexity and phagocytic ability. It appears that where a monocyte lodges has a major influence on its subsequent maturation. For example, the enzymatic activities of pulmonary and peritoneal macrophages are not identical. As might be expected, pulmonary macrophages are more active in aerobic conditions, whereas peritoneal macrophages function primarily in anaerobic conditions. Because of these environmental factors, groups of macrophages are distinguished by their specific functions. These include pulmonary macrophages, osteoclasts, synovial cells, Kupffer cells, Langerhans cells of the skin, microglia cells of the central nervous system, dentritic cells of lymphoid tissues, and others. Tissue macrophages have a long life span. Although usually they are not actively proliferating, many retain the capacity to divide. Their predominant function appears to be maintainance of homeostasis rather than protection against environmental pathogens.

Regardless of their specific functions, the maturation of monocytes into macrophages involves the synthesis of new and often site-specific enzymes, an increase in the endoplasmic reticulum, and increased expression of specific, membrane-associated antigens and receptors.

Monocyte-Macrophage Function

The monocyte-macrophage system plays an essential role in multiple host-defense mechanisms. Functionally, these can be broadly divided into five categories:

1. Initiating an immune response (serving as antigen-presenting cells)
2. Regulating the magnitude of an inflammatory response (secretion of pro- and anti-inflammatory cytokines)
3. Cytotoxic effects:
   a. Phagocytizing and killing of microorganisms
   b. Exerting antiviral and antitumor activities

4. Phagocytizing and degrading worn out cells, cellular debris, and other particulate matter
5. Secreting soluble, biologically active substances other than cytokines

Initiating an Immune Response

In initiating immunologic reactions, monocytes and macrophages have two major functions. The first is to phagocytize and then degrade complex substances into smaller particles, which are able to function as antigens. In most immune reactions, complex proteins and other large molecules do not stimulate a response; small peptide fragments subserve this function. The second function of monocytes and macrophages is to present antigens to responsive lymphocytes. This requires that antigens be localized on the cell's membrane in close association with Class I or II histocompatibility (HLA) antigens (see Chapter 6).

Antigens presented to lymphocytes by macrophages are several thousand times more potent than those in a soluble form. Therefore only a few monocytes or macrophages are required to initiate an immune response. An immune response reaction to the antigen will not occur, however, if the antigen-presenting monocyte/macrophage has HLA determinants different from those of the responsive lymphocyte.

Regulating Inflammation

A related immunologic function of monocytes/macrophages is to regulate the magnitude of an immune response. This function is primarily subserved by the release of soluble mediators, which are capable of either augmenting or suppressing the response. The most important proinflammatory mediators appear to be interleukin-1 (IL-1), tumor necrosis factor alpha (TNF-α), and interleukin-6 (IL-6) (Table 4–3; see also Table 2–3). All three are capable of (1) enhancing local inflammatory reactions; (2) inducing many of the systemic manifestations of inflammation (fever, fatigue, loss of appetite, etc.); (3) promoting the release of acute phase reactants (fibrinogen, C-reactive protein, serum amyloid A protein) from the liver; (4) acting as factors that either directly or indirectly promote hematopoiesis; and (5) potentiating T-cell responses (often in conjugation with other cytokines).

Soluble products of macrophages can also suppress certain immune responses. Among the most potent inhibitors are the **prostaglandins**, particularly **PGE2**. This mediator has inhibitory activities for both lymphocytes and macrophages. Another impor-

Table 4–3 • Cell-Derived Mediators (Cytokines)*

Cytokines	Cellular Source	Principal Activities
TNF-α	Activated macrophages	IL-1–like activities, vascular thrombosis, tumor necrosis
TNF-β	Th1 cells	IL-1–like activities, vascular thrombosis, tumor necrosis
INF-α and β	Macrophages	Antiviral activities, induction of MHC class I antigens, activation of NK cells
INF-γ	Th1 and NK cells	Activation of macrophages, promotion of cell-mediated immunity (Th1 cells), inducing cytoxicity by T cells and NK cells, inhibiting class switching to IgE and IgG1, enhancing expression of MHC class I and class II molecules, antiviral effects
TGF-β	Platelets, macrophages, and lymphocytes	Anti-inflammatory effects, inhibiting proliferation of T cells and macrophages, inducing synthesis of extracellular matrix proteins

*Cytokines are protein factors produced by various cells. They mediate and regulate immune and inflammatory reactions.

tant negative regulatory factor is transforming growth factor beta (**TGF-β**). This regulator, which is also synthesized by T and B lymphocytes, platelets, and other cells, has antiproliferative properties that affect several types of cells, including lymphocytes and macrophages. It also suppresses production of numerous cytokines and reduces expression of class II HLA antigens and certain cellular receptors, including those for IL-1. TGF-β also possesses proinflammatory activities. It can be a chemoattractant for neutrophils and monocytes and stimulate expression of adhesion molecules.

Cytotoxic Effects

Macrophages ingest and kill microorganisms by processes similar to those of neutrophils. Macrophages are the primary defense against intracellular pathogens including Mycobacterium tuberculosis, many bacteria, virtually all protozoa and fungi, and many viruses.

A key feature of macrophage killing is cell activation. Soluble products of T lymphocytes, particularly γ interferon, convert resting macrophages into cells that can actively kill intracellular organisms, and exhibit lytic activities for specific tumor cells.

One of the best models for understanding the relationship between intracellular organisms, macrophage activation, and T-lymphocyte function is the in vivo infection of mice with Listeria monocytogenes. After infection these organisms are phagocytized by macrophages, primarily in the liver and spleen. In the absence of a specific T-cell immune response, the bacteria persist within the cytoplasm of these phagocytic cells for indefinite periods. Once a T-cell response has been initiated, however, γ interferon activates the infected macrophages and rapidly converts them into efficient killers. The microorganisms are quickly and completely eliminated.

In this sequence, macrophage activation is a nonspecific event. Following activation, these cells kill virtually any intracellular pathogen. For example, γ interferon elicited from tuberculin-sensitized T lymphocytes exposed to tuberculin antigen can transform quiescent macrophages infected with Listeria into cells capable of killing that microorganism.

Macrophages have both antiviral and antitumor activities. One mechanism that protects against viral invasion is the synthesis and secretion of α interferon (the form produced by leukocytes, primarily monocytes and macrophages). Alpha interferon induces macrophages to increase their expression of class II MHC antigens and receptors for the Fc portion of IgG. It also has antiproliferative activities, inhibiting the growth of lymphocytes, bone marrow precursors, and certain tumor cells (see Table 4–3).

Housekeeping Functions

Macrophages ingest and degrade cellular debris such as senescent neutrophils. They also secrete proteases, which help to liquefy and eliminate an inflammatory exudate.

Secreting Growth Factors

Another major function of macrophages in the host defense system is to elaborate hematopoietic growth factors. Macrophages are a major source of the growth factors G-CSF, M-CSF, and GM-CSF. Thus they serve as an important control for the production of new cells from the bone marrow. Several other interleukins are also produced by macrophages, as are other compounds that can affect the status of both the phagocytic and immune systems.

Eosinophils

Because of the intense staining of their granules with acid dyes, eosinophils are among the most colorful of all the leukocytes. (Ehrlich named them after Eos, the ancient Greek goddess of the dawn.) These cells are slightly larger than neutrophils and generally have a bilobular nucleus. Normally, they comprise only 1% to 3% of the circulating white cells. **Eosinophilia**, an increase in the number of eosinophils in the blood, is seen in a variety of allergic, parasitic, and immunologic disorders. Its presence may be an important diagnostic clue to many systemic disorders.

Eosinophils share many developmental characteristics with neutrophils. They arise from the multipotential myeloid progenitors, which can differentiate into eosinophilic precursors, detectable in culture as eosinophilic colony-forming cells. The growth of eosinophils is highly dependent on the cytokine IL-5. Eosinophils have a marrow transit time of 2 to 6 days. Like neutrophils, mature eosinophils are terminally differentiated cells, lacking the capacity for further proliferative expansion. They circulate in the blood with an average life span of 6 to 12 hours and enter the tissues, where they appear to have a life span of a few days.

The functions of eosinophils are poorly understood. These cells appear to be able to both enhance and suppress inflammatory responses. They are capable of phagocytosis, but this may not be their major function. Studies suggest that eosinophils can attach to antibody- or complement-coated particles and, through a complex process, release the contents of granules that, in turn, can kill selected parasites. Thus one of the major functions of eosinophils appears to be mediating host defenses against helminthic and other parasitic infections.

The number of eosinophils is also increased in a number of allergic or hypersensitivity conditions, in certain neoplastic diseases, and as a component of myeloproliferative diseases. In clinical practice, probably the most common cause of an eosinophilia is a hypersensitivity reaction to a drug. **Idiopathic hypereosinophilia** is a rare condition characterized by a persistent elevation of blood eosinophils and tissue damage, primarily to the heart and the central nervous system. The cause of this disorder is not known; it has been speculated that it may be related to excessive production of IL-5. Hypereosinophilia tends to run a chronic course, but it has a high mortality rate if untreated. In most patients it can be controlled by corticosteroids, cytotoxic drugs, or α-interferon.

Basophils

Basophils are the rarest but one of the most distinctive types of leukocyte in the peripheral blood. Morphologically, they contain prominent basophilic granules, which are often dense enough to obscure the nucleus of the cell. These granules contain many soluble mediators of inflammation such as histamine, the anticoagulant heparin, kallikreins, eosinophil chemotactic factors, and leukotrienes. Functionally, basophils are key mediators of immediate hypersensitivity reactions, which are initiated by binding of IgE to specific receptors on the basophils. This reaction induces the external release of intracellular granules.

Functionally, tissue **mast cells** are closely related to basophils. Like basophils, they have prominent cytoplasmic granules that contain similar mediators of inflammation. These cells appear to be derived from precursors in the marrow. In contrast to blood basophils, mast cells have a long life span and are capable of local proliferation. Tissue mast cells may arise from a separate cell lineage rather than from the transformation of basophils.

5 Lymphocytes and the Immune System

Lymphocytes, the second most numerous type of white cells in the peripheral blood, are essential components of a functioning immune defense system. Their primary activity is reacting with antigens, thereby initiating a series of events leading to a specific immune response. It is not surprising that diseases affecting lymphocytes frequently manifest themselves as either an inability to protect the individual from environmental pathogens (**an immune deficiency syndrome**) or the development of immune responses directed at self-antigen (**autoimmunity**).

Based on differences in their functional activities, lymphocytes constitute a heterogeneous population of cells, but the functional groups cannot be distinguished morphologically. Nearly all blood lymphocytes (more than 95%) appear as small cells with scant amounts of cytoplasm and a lack of distinctive morphologic features. These small lymphocytes can be considered resting or quiescent cells. When they are exposed to an appropriate antigen or **mitogen** (a substance that causes a cell to enter mitosis), they are transformed into rapidly proliferating cells. Intermixed with these small lymphocytes are a few medium or large lymphocytes. These are cells with more abundant cytoplasm and less-condensed nuclear chromatin. They are believed to be derived from small lymphocytes and are considered to be cells in the process of responding to an immunologic stimulus.

The major functional groups of lymphocytes include:

- Those derived from the thymus (thymic-dependent or **T cells**), which are primarily responsible for cell-mediated immunity
- Bone marrow lymphocytes (**B cells**), which can synthesize specific antibodies and are themselves the precursors of plasma cells
- Natural killer cells (**NK cells**), which are able to kill certain tumor cells and virally infected target cells.

The T-cell population has been further subdivided into those considered to function primarily as helper or inducer cells (**helper/inducer T lymphocytes**) and those that are antigen-specific cytotoxic cells (**cytotoxic/cytolytic T lymphocytes**).

The blood pool represents only a minor fraction of the total body pool of lymphoid cells. Most can be found in organized lymphoid tissues such as lymph nodes, spleen, and Peyer's patches in the intestines. Unlike neutrophils, lymphocytes can both enter and leave the circulation, a process termed **recirculation.** This is an important property because it permits the dissemination of immunologic information throughout the body. Despite this complex circulatory pattern, however, the entire lymphoid system is normally maintained in equilibrium; cells leaving the circulation are balanced by an equal input of lymphocytes from the tissue pools. In a steady state, the number of circulating lymphocytes remains relatively constant.

The **lymphoid system** is subdivided into primary and secondary organs. The primary organs include the bone marrow and the thymus; these are sites for the production of naïve lymphocytes (immunologically competent cells that have not been exposed to antigen). The secondary organs are the lymph nodes, which are widely distributed throughout the body; the spleen; and the mucosa-associated lymphoid tissues (MALT). These are sites for immune reactions and for the generation of memory/effector lymphocytes. The secondary lymphoid organs are interconnected to each other through both blood vessels and a series of low-pressure lymphatic vascular channels (**lymphatics**). Lymphatics contain an ultrafiltrate of blood in which is suspended a virtually pure population of lymphocytes.

Functional Division of the Immune System

Because lymphocytes are the primary effectors of immune responses, an appreciation of the general types of immune responses is essential for an understanding of the physiology and pathology of these cells. There are two general types of immune responses: **cell-mediated reactions** and **humoral reactions**. Cell-mediated reactions occur only at the site of antigen deposition and require direct cell contact between the inciting antigen and the effector T lymphocyte. Depending on the antigen, cell-mediated reactions may entail the direct killing of tumor cells or those infected with specific viruses (**cytotoxicity**) or may involve the release of soluble mediators that recruit and activate nonspecific effector cells such as macrophages.

Cytotoxic/cytolytic T cells are active only if they have been previously sensitized to the antigenic target and if there is compatibility between HLA determinants on the antigen-presenting cells and their receptors on the effector T cells. The process of cell-mediated cytotoxicity is not restricted to T cells, however. NK cells are also potent cytolytic elements, which appear to serve as the first line of defense against tumors or virally infected cells. Unlike the cytotoxic/cytolytic T cells, NK cells can effect responses in the absence of either prior exposure to the target antigen or HLA compatibility.

The other major component of the immune defense system is **humoral immunity**. This group of reactions is effected by the synthesis and secretion of proteins called **antibodies**, which are specifically modified to react with the inciting antigen. As a group, antibodies are collectively referred to as **immunoglobulins**. Although cell-mediated reactions require direct contact between the T-effector cell and the antigen, humoral immune reactions, once established, can occur at sites distant from the cells synthesizing the antibody. The effectors of humoral immunity are B lymphocytes and their progeny, plasma cells.

A prime function of the immune defense system is to protect against environmental pathogens. Each immune component is dominant in the resistance to specific classes of infectious agents. The elimination of encapsulated pyogenic bacteria, such as *pneumococci* and *Haemophilus influenzae*, is highly dependent on the presence of antibodies specific for antigenic determinants on these organisms. Patients with disorders characterized by defective antibody production are particularly vulnerable to these bacterial infections. By contrast, cell-mediated immunity is the principal defense mechanism against intracellular organisms, including many bacteria and most fungi, protozoa, and viruses. The importance of this kind of immunity is particularly illustrated by the vast array of complicating infections occurring in patients with the acquired immune deficiency syndrome (AIDS). These individuals have a profound defect in cell-mediated immune responses, leaving them

Table 5–1 • Major Activities of Humoral and Cell-Mediated Immunity

Humoral Immunity

Elimination of encapsulated bacteria

Neutralization of soluble toxins; viral protection (incubation phase)

Transplantation rejection reactions (hyperacute reaction)

Immunologically related disease (autoimmune blood dyscrasia, "toxic complex" diseases, allergic disorders)

Cell-Mediated Immunity

Resistance against intracellular pathogens (many bacteria, most viruses, protozoa, fungi)

Transplantation rejection reactions (acute and chronic reaction)

Tumor immunity

Autoimmunity (role not well defined)

Contact dermatitis

---

highly susceptible to infections by many intracellular organisms (e.g., toxoplasmosis, cryptococcus, tuberculosis, etc.).

In addition to protecting against pathogenic microorganisms, both immune mechanisms serve several other functions, which are summarized in Table 5–1.

Most antigens elicit both a cell-mediated and a humoral immune reaction, and studies have shown that there is a complex cellular interaction between different types of lymphocytes in generating both types of responses. For example, both T cells and antigen-presenting cells are essential for many B-cell responses. As a result of their activity, the B-cell population becomes activated, secretes specific immunoglubulins, and terminally differentiates into plasma cells.

Development of the Lymphoid System

T-Cell Development

Lymphocytes initially arise from the same pluripotential stem cells that give rise to myeloid elements (Figure 5–1). As previously mentioned, this primitive stem cell is believed to be the precursor of two more restricted types of progenitor cells: one that gives rise to hematopoietic elements and one that is a precursor of T, B, and NK lymphocytes.

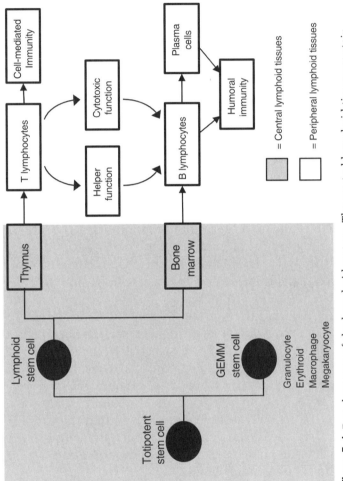

Figure 5–1. Development of the lymphoid system. The central lymphoid tissues contain immunologically immature cells; the peripheral tissues are populated by lymphocytes capable of effecting an immune response (competent cells). Despite the apparent independent development of T and B cells, the two systems are highly interdependent.

Progenitors for T lymphocytes originate in the bone marrow and other primitive hematopoietic tissues and migrate via the blood to the outer cortex of the thymus. At this site the cells undergo extensive proliferative expansion and a complex process of maturation. Concomitantly with these maturation processes, primitive T cells migrate toward the medullary region of the thymus. One of the striking characteristics of thymopoiesis is that it is a very selective process. Most of the cells die within the thymus. Fewer than 1% emerge from this organ to seed peripheral lymphoid tissues.

T-cell maturation within the thymus requires a coordinated series of events during which the cell rearranges the gene segments coding for the T-cell receptor (TCR). This process establishes the specificity of the cell for a single antigenic determinant. Antigenic specificity is determined by the amino acid sequence of the variable regions of the T-cell receptor.

The genetic process by which each variable region of the receptor acquires specificity is termed **rearrangement**. Pre-T cells, as well as all somatic cells, contain the gene segments coding for these polypeptide chains in a "germline" configuration, a complex structure containing groups of gene segments coding for different portions of the variable region. Each of these groups contains multiple exons, each capable of coding for a specific amino acid sequence. The gene segment groupings are designated the variable (V), the diversity (D), and the joining (J) regions. Rearrangement entails the selection and isolation of a single exon from each region (Figure 5–2), followed by splicing the selected exons together to form the genetic sequence coding for amino acids of the variable region. Thus, one V-region gene segment is joined to one gene segment from the D region and one from the J region to code for a specific sequence. The newly formed gene segment for the variable region then combines with the gene segment for the constant region, yielding a DNA sequence, termed a **rearranged gene**, which codes for the entire polypeptide chain.

The T-cell receptor, present on the cell membrane of immunologically competent T cells, is a heterodimer consisting of two polypeptide chains, an α chain and a β chain, linked by disulfide bonds. Each chain is composed of a variable region and one or more constant regions. The variable region defines the chain's ability to bind to a single antigenic determinant. The rearranged T-cell receptor gene is transcribed into a protein, which localizes to cell membrane on immunologically competent T lymphocytes. It appears

Germline Configuration

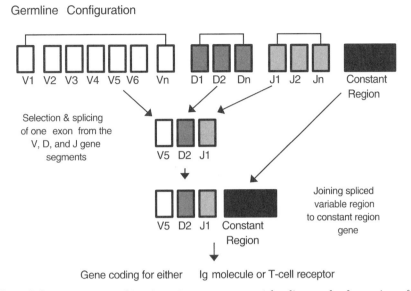

Figure 5–2. Genetic recombinations (rearrangements) leading to the formation of the variable region for one chain of the T-cell receptor. Before the recombination, the receptor gene segments are in the germline configuration and each segment contains several exons. Each segment codes for one of the three specific regions, V, D, and J. Antigen specificity is determined by selecting one exon coding for a V region and joining it to an exon coding for the D region and one for the J region. Based on this model, it is possible for a finite number of genes to code for virtually all of the antigen specificities that an individual will encounter in his or her lifetime. A similar selection process is also used by B lymphocytes to code for the variable regions of immunoglobulin molecules

that the intracytoplasmic tail of the receptor protein is too short to transmit signals arising from antigenic binding to the receptor. Rather, this signaling function results from a second membrane-associated protein, the CD3 complex (Figure 5–3). (See "Identification of Lymphocyte Subsets" later in this chapter.) The CD3 complex is expressed in all immunologically competent T lymphocytes.

In addition to αβ T-cell receptors, there is a minor population of peripheral T cells that express an alternate receptor, the γδ receptor. To date, the function of these γδ receptor cells has not been fully defined.

Normal thymic development can be followed by a series of changes in the expression of specific T-cell-related antigens (Figure 5–4). The most primitive thymocytes express on their membrane a group of pan-T-cell antigens, CD2, CD5, and CD7.

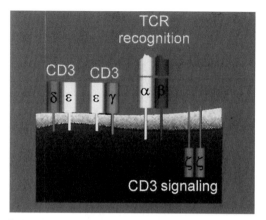

Figure 5–3. This schematic representation of the T-cell receptor (TCR)/CD3 complex shows the T-cell receptor's α and β chains with their antigen recognition site in close contact with the CD3 molecule. The CD3 molecule is composed of three dimerized chains, the δε and εγ heterodimers with prominent external receptor components, and the ζζ homodimer with a prominent intracellular signaling component.

They lack the CD3 antigen (the antigen associated with the T-cell receptor) and those that mark for the helper/inducer (CD4) or cytotoxic/cytolytic phenotype (CD8), sometimes referred to as "suppressor" cells (see page 84). During an intermediate stage of maturation, thymocytes initially co-express both the CD4 and CD8 antigens and are called "double-positive cells," CD4$^+$ and CD8$^+$; subsequently, the cells segregate into two mutually exclusive populations, each of which expresses either the CD4 or CD8 antigen, but not both. This segregation is associated with the acquisition of membrane CD3. In patients with T-cell acute lymphoblastic leukemia, the stage of maturation arrest can be determined by examining leukemic cells for their expression of these antigens (see Figure 5–4).

Two facets of thymus cell maturation are important. First, the thymus is primarily functional during fetal life. In humans, the peripheral T-cell system is almost fully developed at birth and does not require a significant input of new cells for its maintenance. Thus it is possible to surgically remove the thymus without causing severe immunologic failure. By contrast, failure of the thymus to form during fetal life is associated with a severe T-cell immunodeficiency (DiGeorge's syndrome), which usually results in death during infancy as a consequence of repeated infections.

The second facet of thymic maturation is that the development of mature T cells appears to be controlled both by humoral

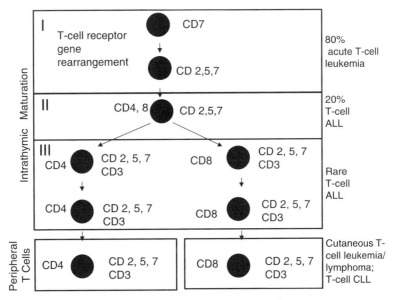

Figure 5–4. Changes in the phenotype of thymocytes with maturation. Anatomically, the most primitive thymocytes are located in the outer cortex of the thymus. As cells mature, they migrate toward the medulla. Thymopoiesis is very selective; fewer than 1% of the cells in the thymus ever mature into immunologically competent T cells. Thymocytes develop their surface antigen expression in stages, from early thymocytes (stage I) through intermediate and late thymocytes (stages II and III). T-cell leukemias of different types may be derived from the thymocytes of each of the stages. Although T cells do not express surface CD3 until stage III of intrathymic development, this antigen may be found in the cytoplasm much earlier.

factors synthesized by its stromal elements and by the presence of cells bearing MHC antigens. Several soluble factors have been isolated, characterized, and purified from the thymus, but none of these isolates has yet been able to restore T-cell competency in immunodeficient patients.

B-Cell Maturation

The initial stages of the maturation of stem cells into immunologically competent B lymphocytes appear to occur primarily within the bone marrow. Like the T cells, B cells arise from pluripotential stem cells. The earliest pre-B cells have been identified by their expression of a specific pan–B-cell antigen, CD19. The maturation process is subsequently characterized by an orderly acquisition and loss of antigens (Figure 5–5). After the appearance of CD19, the cells acquire CD10, a determinant that has been called the common

Antigen-independent　　　　**Antigen-dependent**

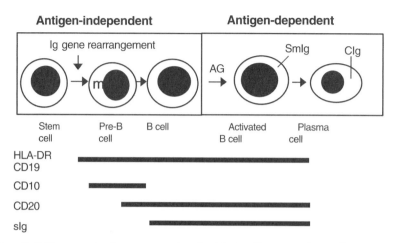

Figure 5–5. Phenotypic changes associated with B-cell maturation. All events occurring before acquisition of surface immunoglobulins are independent of antigenic exposure. Plasma cells do not express surface membrane immunoglobulin (SmIg) but do contain cytoplasmic immunoglobulin (CIg). AG = antigen; Ig = immunoglobulin.

acute lymphoblastic leukemic antigen (CALLA) because of its presence on many acute lymphoblastic leukemic cells. The next stage is the appearance of another pan–B-cell antigen, CD20. The last stage in the maturation of pre-B cells is characterized by the appearance of the heavy chains of IgM immunoglobulin, μ, in the cell's cytoplasm. These heavy chains are not found in association with light chains, nor are they expressed on the cell's membrane.

The pre-B cell then matures into an immunologically competent B cell. This process results in the expression of a complete immunoglobulin on the cell's membrane (surface membrane immunoglobulin [SmIg]) and a loss of both the CD10 antigen and detectable intracytoplasmic μ heavy chains. The membrane-bound immunoglobulin constitutes the cell's antigen receptor. The sequence of antigen acquisition and loss can be used clinically to define the stage of maturation arrest of a pre–B-cell acute leukemia. The final stage of B-cell maturation is the plasma cell (described later).

As in the T cell, the immunoglobulin genes of the pre-B cell undergo a rearrangement process (see Figure 5–2). Immature pre-B cells and all other somatic cells contain the genes coding for the immunoglobulin molecules in a germline configuration, with multiple exons coding for V, D, and J gene segments of the variable region. As with T cells, during the early stage of the development of pre-B cells these gene segments undergo a rearrangement process, which entails the splicing and joining of one V exon to one exon from the D region and the one from the J region. This rearranged variable gene segment is then combined with the gene segment that codes for the constant region of either the heavy or light chain genes. Because of this recombination process, an almost infinite number of antibody-combining sites can be generated. As discussed later, the antigen-combining site consists of the variable regions of both the light and heavy chains. This antigen-specific complex has been termed the **idiotype**.

Lymphocyte Responses to Antigens

Immunologically competent lymphocytes undergo a coordinated series of morphologic and biochemical events when responding to a specific antigenic challenge. Before this contact, these cells exist as small, intermitotic lymphocytes.

T Cells

In the T-cell system, the initiation of an immune response depends upon the binding of antigen, presented on the surface of an antigen-presenting cell, to the T-cell receptor. To initiate a response, the antigen is presented in conjunction with the MHC complex; the CD4 and CD8 molecules on T cells serve as co-stimulatory molecules. CD4 is a receptor for class II MHC molecules and CD8 for class I molecules.

This interaction induces a series of events, which can be divided into five interrelated stages:

1. Early signal transduction
2. Transcriptional activation of genes
3. Expression of new cell membrane molecules
4. Secretion of cytokines
5. Induction of mitotic activity

The early activation events occur within seconds after an antigen binds to the T-cell receptor (Figure 5–6). The initial event is activation of G proteins, and the phospholipase-C-associated hydrolysis of phosphatidyl inositol biphosphate (PIP_2). This leads to the hydrolytic release of two second messengers, diacylglycerol (DAG) and inositol triphosphate (IP_3). DAG, a membrane-bound

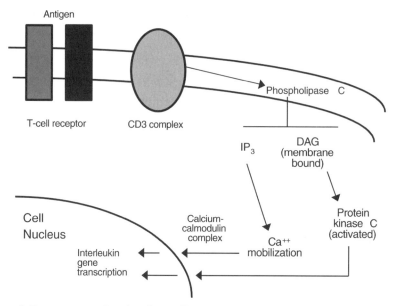

Figure 5–6. Events associated with T-cell activation. Binding of antigen to the T-cell receptor stimulates the hydrolysis by phospholipase C of PIP_2 to form membrane-bound diacylglycerol (DAG) and cytoplasmic inositol triphosphate (IP_3). The DAG activates protein kinase C (PKC), and IP_3 mobilizes calcium (Ca^{++}) from cytoplasmic stores. The Ca^{++} combines with and activates a regulatory protein, calmodulin. Both PKC and the Ca^{++}-calmodulin complex activate transcription factors in the nucleus, activating genes that are responsible for interleukin synthesis and receptor expression. As discussed, one of the most important interleukins is IL-2; IL-2 and its receptor are responsible for T-cell replication.

compound, activates protein kinase C (PKC), and IP_3 causes the release of cytoplasmic calcium (Ca^{++}), which combines with and activates a regulatory protein, calmodulin, causing calcium-dependent phosphorylation reactions. Both PKC and the Ca^{++}-calmodulin complex help to initiate reactions leading to activation of factors that, in turn, will activate genes inducing production of RNA, which will lead to cytokine production and cytokine receptor expression. Antigen binding to the T-cell receptor also activates tyrosine kinases, which help to augment this activation process. In the T-cell system, one of the principal cytokines is interleukin 2 (IL-2). The genes for transcribing IL-2 and those coding for the receptor for IL-2 are activated at the same time, leading to receptor expression on the T-cell membrane. The binding of IL-2 to its receptor induces clonal T-cell proliferation.

These biochemical events are associated with a series of morphologic changes in the lymphocyte (Figure 5–7). Stimulated cells appear to dedifferentiate, assuming a more immature morphologic appearance. They show increased amounts of basophilic cytoplasm, a larger nucleus with less condensed nuclear chromatin, and often the presence of discernible nucleoli. Morphologically, these antigen-activated cells are considered to be transformed or dedifferentiated cells. Such cells undergo repetitive mitotic divisions leading to the formation of a clone of daughter cells, each programmed to respond to the same inciting antigen. After proliferation, the daughter cells mature into immunologic effectors, which again assume the appearance of small lymphocytes.

In effecting a response, the CD4$^+$ helper/inducer cells act primarily by synthesizing and secreting cytokines that act on other cells. By contrast, CD8$^+$ cells are directly cytotoxic for target cells (tumor cells or virally infected cells) that express the inciting antigen on their cell membrane. Recent studies suggest that there are two subsets of T helper (Th) cells, designated Th1 and Th2. The Th1 cells synthesize and secrete IL-2 and gamma interferon, which itself is a potent activator of macrophages. The Th1 cells are primarily

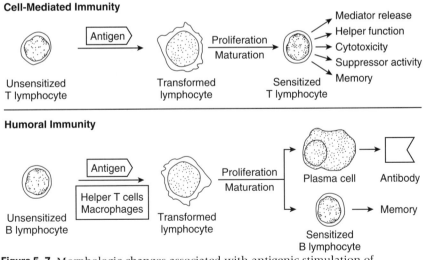

Figure 5–7. Morphologic changes associated with antigenic stimulation of immunologically competent lymphocytes. These changes include dedifferentiation into more immature forms, active cell proliferation, and final maturation of daughter cells into immune effectors. A proportion of the daughter cells do not participate in the immediate reaction, but rather reenter the pool of recirculating lymphocytes to serve as memory T and B cells.

involved in effecting cell-mediated responses. Th2 cells act as primary mediators for humoral immune responses by releasing interleukins, including IL-4, IL-6, IL-10, and IL-13.

T cells may also exhibit suppressor activity. At one time, a definite suppressor subset was believed to exist in the $CD8^+$ subset, but no such definite subset has been identified. Nevertheless, by convention, $CD8^+$ cells continue to be spoken of as **suppressor cells** and the CD4:CD8 ratio is often referred to as the helper:suppressor ratio.

In addition, some of the T cells derived from the original contact with the antigen return to the pool of recirculating lymphocytes to serve as memory cells. These cells are already programmed to respond to the inciting antigen, so that on reexposure they can react more rapidly, giving a secondary or anamnestic immune response.

B Cells

The initial responses of B lymphocytes to antigens are quite similar to those occurring in T lymphocytes. The antigen receptor on a B cell is an antibody with specificity for the inciting antigen. Typically, the antibody is of the IgM isotype; on some B cells, IgM and IgD are co-expressed. When the two antibody isotypes are present, they share a single antigenic specificity.

Like the T cell, each B lymphocyte is programmed to respond to a single antigen. In many B-cell reactions, the response requires that the antigen initially induce a T helper cell response, which provides stimulatory interleukins (as mentioned above) capable of inducing B-cell transformation, proliferation, and terminal differentiation. The biochemical changes that accompany B lymphocyte activation are similar to those described for T cells (see Figure 5–7).

One of the major differences between the two systems is the final effectors. In the B-cell system, these are specialized cells called **plasma cells**, which are highly efficient in synthesizing and secreting large quantities of antibodies specific for the inciting antigen. These cells do not express SmIg but do contain cytoplasmic immunoglobulin (CIg) (see Figure 5–5). Terminally differentiated plasma cells are considered to be "end-stage" cells; they are unable to proliferate. A subset of B lymphocytes responding to the initial antigenic challenge seem to revert back to small lymphocytes and serve as B memory cells.

Natural Killer Cells

Most of the other lymphocytes in the blood belong to the class of cytotoxic cells called **natural killer (NK) cells**. Morphologically, these cells are often slightly larger than typical small lymphocytes. Their cytoplasm is more abundant and may contain large azurophilic granules. NK cells are cytolytic for both tumor cells and virally infected cells. Unlike cytotoxic T lymphocytes, NK cells can kill targets in the absence of prior immune sensitization and despite HLA differences. Because of their ability to kill without prior sensitization, NK cells are thought to be the first line of defense against both microorganisms and tumors.

Identification of Lymphocyte Subsets

Functional populations of lymphocytes cannot be identified by routine morphologic criteria. Conventional microscopy cannot discern any features that reliably differentiate T, B, and NK cells. By virtue of differences in their membrane constituents, however, immunophenotyping permits the recognition of functionally different types of lymphocytes. In this process, an antibody is prepared against a unique cell membrane determinant. The antibody is then labeled with a visible dye, which allows for its identification. The most common labels are dyes that can be visualized with fluorescence microscopy. An antigen-specific monoclonal antibody will selectively react with all cells bearing this determinant, and cells of interest can be positively identified and enumerated.

In most clinical laboratories, this process has been automated. The number of cells binding a specific antibody are detected electronically. The instrument used for this detection is a **flow cytometer**. This type of analysis has proven invaluable in the management of patients with immune deficiency syndromes such as AIDS and in determining the cellular origins of neoplastic leukemic and lymphoma cells.

Initial studies with immunophenotyping were complicated by the presence of a bewildering assortment of names applied to various antibodies reacting with the same antigen. To provide a uniform system of nomenclature, it was decided that all antibodies that react with an epitope of the same membrane determinant would be grouped together and given a single "cluster of differentiation" (CD) number. Cells bearing the specific determinant were then designated by this CD number. A list of some commonly used CD numbers is shown in Table 5–2.

T cells are generally identified by the presence of the CD3 antigen, the polypeptide associated with the T-cell receptor. This antigen is lacking from other types of lymphocytes. As previously

Table 5–2 • Common CD Designations Used for Cell Identification

CD Number	Cell Type
T Cells	
CD2	Pan-T cell
CD5	Pan-T cell; subset of B cells
CD7	Pan-T cell
CD3	Antigen on all mature (immunocompetent) T cells; associated with T-cell receptor
CD4	T helper/inducer subset; reacts with class II MHC antigens
CD8	T cytotoxic/cytolytic subset; reacts with class I MHC antigens
B Cells	
CD19	Pan-B cell
CD20	Pan-B cell
CD10	Stage-specific antigen present on pre-B cells and acute lymphoblastic leukemic cells (also called CALLA)
NK Cells	
CD16	Fc receptor
CD56	NK cells
Stem Cells	
CD34	Pluripotential stem cells and progenitors
Myeloid Cells	
CD33	Early myeloid cells
CD13	Panmyeloid cells
CD14	Monocytes
HLA-DR*	B cells, myeloid blasts, and monocytes. Not present on promyelocytes and later-stage myeloid cells.

*HLA-DR antigen has not been assigned a CD number, but it is a specific cell marker nevertheless.

described, the peripheral T-cell compartment is further subdivided into two mutually exclusive subsets, the CD4$^+$ or T helper/inducer cells and the CD8$^+$ or T cytotoxic/cytolytic cells. Before acquisition of immunologic competency, developing T cells do not express the CD3 antigen on the surface. Pan–T-cell antigens, including the CD2, CD5, and CD7 antigens, can be detected both on mature T lymphocytes and on thymocytes.

Similarly, B lymphocytes can be positively identified by the presence of membrane-associated immunoglobulins. B cells are also known to possess certain lineage-specific antigens; antibodies to two of these antigens, CD19 and CD20, are widely used for B-cell quantitation. Both of these antigens are present on early pre-B cells and persist until a cell is stimulated by an antigen and undergoes terminal differentiation into a plasma cell.

NK cells are negative for both CD3 and surface immunoglobulins, but they do react with certain antibodies such as CD16 and CD56.

In normal blood, 60% to 85% of the circulating lymphocytes are T cells. Of these, about two thirds are $CD4^+$ cells and one third are $CD8^+$ cells (a ratio of approximately 2:1). About 3% to 27% of the lymphocytes are B cells, and 3% to 19% are NK cells.

Lymphocyte Life Span and Circulation

Unlike neutrophils, the vast majority of blood lymphocytes are classified as **recirculating cells;** they are able to leave and reenter the bloodstream. This process is essential for the dissemination of immunologic information throughout the body. Furthermore, this recirculation process is not a random migration of lymphocytes but rather one in which cells "home" primarily to environments similar to those in which they initially encountered antigen. Thus, lymphocytes that have been exposed to or programmed by antigens in peripheral lymphoid tissues tend to preferentially migrate to the lymph nodes and to the skin. Lymphocytes programmed in the mesenteric lymph nodes, on the other hand, recirculate primarily to the MALT (Figure 5–8).

In recent years we have learned more about the mechanisms involved in lymphoid recirculation. Molecular mechanisms similar to those involved in neutrophil adhesion and migration also seem to apply to lymphocytes. Although somewhat different adhesion molecules are involved, there is an initial loose adhesion or rolling motion of lymphocytes over endothelial venule cells. The lymphocytes then become firmly attached to endothelial cells and finally migrate between the endothelial cells into the tissues. In the extravascular spaces lymphocytes can migrate to regional lymph nodes, enter efferent lymph vessels, and ultimately return to the blood via the thoracic duct and other connections between the lymph vessels and the blood. The transit times of lymphocytes in the blood are rather short, estimated to be ½ hour to 2 hours. The time spent in lymphatic tissues is also short, usually 1 to 2 days. Thus, during the life span of a long-lived lymphocyte, the cell

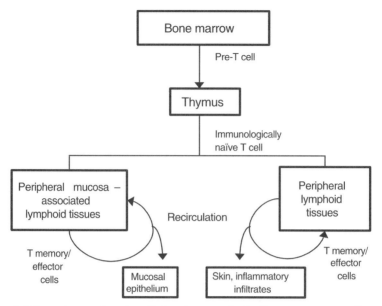

Figure 5–8. Lymphocyte homing. Naïve, immunologically competent T cells emigrate from the thymus and randomly migrate to either the mucosa-associated lymphoid tissues (MALT) or the other peripheral lymphoid tissues. In these secondary organs, they acquire specific adhesion molecules that program them to recirculate specifically to the type of lymphoid organs where they received their initial programming. T cells initially conditioned in peripheral lymphoid tissues can also migrate into the skin or areas of inflammation. MALT-programmed cells also migrate into mucosal epithelial surfaces.

enters and leaves the circulation several thousand times. Lymphocyte recirculation is diagrammatically depicted in Figure 5–9.

Virgin lymphocytes (those that have not yet been exposed to antigen) initially migrate to the secondary lymphoid organs. They do not show a preference for a particular type of secondary lymphoid tissue, and they do not efficiently migrate from their sites of production (thymus, bone marrow) to extralymphoid sites such as the skin or mucosal epithelium. By contrast, memory/effector lymphocytes, cells that have been programmed to respond to an antigen, have a different migratory pattern. They can enter tertiary lymphoid sites such as the skin and mucosal epithelium. They are also able to localize to sites of antigen deposition (see Figure 5–8).

The selective homing behavior of memory lymphocytes is achieved by differential expression of adhesion molecules. The surface molecules mediating organ-specific binding of lymphocytes to high endothelial venules (vessels with plump endothelial

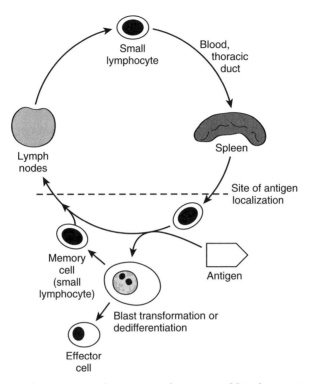

Figure 5–9. Lymphocyte recirculation. Lymphocytes, unlike phagocytic cells, can both enter and leave the circulation. The initial phases of this process closely resemble the migration of neutrophils from the blood into the tissues; lymphocytes migrate between the junctions of high endothelial venule cells. The migratory process is interrupted when the lymphocyte encounters an appropriate antigenic stimulus. Recirculation is an important process for disseminating immunologic information throughout the body.

lining cells) have been called **lymphocyte homing receptors** and their counter-receptors on the endothelial surface are called **addressins.** Four addressins have been immunologically or molecularly identified:

1. **GlyCAM-1** (glycosylated cell adhesion molecule-1, also called peripheral node addressin or PNAd) is involved in lymphocyte adhesion to the high endothelial venules (HEV) in peripheral lymph nodes. L selectin is the lymphocyte homing receptor that mediates lymphocyte adhesion.
2. **MAdCAM-1** (mucosal addressin cell adhesion molecule-1) is involved in lymphocyte adhesion to HEV expressed in mucosal lymph nodes, mediated by an integrin, $\alpha 4/\beta 7$.

3. **Synovial addressin** (currently identified by monoclonal antibodies only) is expressed on HEV in inflamed synovium.

4. **E selectin** is involved in the recruitment of memory T cells to skin during inflammatory dermatoses such as contact dermatitis. Cutaneous lymphocyte-associated antigen (CLA), a sialyated structure on $CD4^+$ memory lymphocytes, is the receptor that binds to E selectin.

The migratory pattern of circulating lymphocytes may be modified during antigen-induced proliferation, partly because the expression of lymphocyte homing receptors changes. L selectin is downregulated on normal cells during proliferation and subsequently is reexpressed on some memory cells, but not all. Conversely, the lymphocyte homing receptor CLA is acquired by a subset of T cells during conversion into memory cells.

The turnover rate of peripheral blood T cells is extremely slow. It has been estimated that the average interval between T-cell divisions is approximately 3 years, and some cells can survive for more than 10 years without dividing. This long life span is one of the reasons why immunologic memory persists; cells programmed to recognize antigens seen in the remote past potentially can remain in a quiescent phase for the life span of the individual.

Immunoglobulins

Immunoglobulins (Ig) is a term collectively used to describe **serum antibodies**, a heterogeneous group of proteins, each specifically modified to react with a particular antigen. The major source of antibodies is plasma cells. Small amounts are also produced by B lymphocytes. All antibodies of the same type that are specific for a single antigen are derived from a single clone of cells. Thus a clone represents a population of cells, all with a single common precursor. Each cell in a B-cell clone is programmed to respond by elaborating the same antibody.

Structure

All immunoglobulins have a common structure consisting of four polypeptide chains: two identical heavy chains and two identical light chains (Figure 5–10). These are held together by disulfide bonds. The light chains are common to all types of immunoglobulin and the heavy chain determines the class specificity of the immunoglobulin. Based on differences in the heavy chains, immunoglobulins are subdivided into five classes or **isotypes,** shown in order

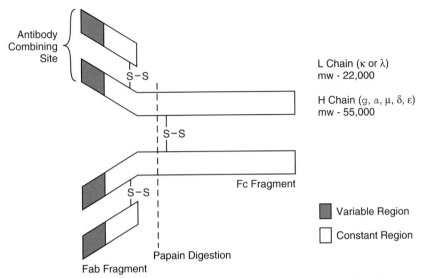

Figure 5–10. Structure of the basic immunoglobulin subunit. Each subunit has two antibody-combining sites, composed of the variable regions of both the light chains (VL) and heavy chains (VH). The remaining portions of both the light and heavy chains are called the constant (C) regions. Those pertaining to the heavy chain are designated CH1, CH2, and CH3, representing three constant domains of the heavy chain. CL represents the constant region of the light chain.

of decreasing concentration in Table 5–3. IgG, IgA, IgD, and IgE consist of monomers of this molecule; IgM is a pentameter that consists of five monomeric units bound together by a polypeptide known as the J chain. Dimers of IgA also occur.

    There are two types of light chains, kappa (κ) and lambda (λ). Each immunoglobulin molecule consists of two identical light chains, either κ or λ, and two identical heavy chains. Both the light and heavy chains consist of regions designated variable and

Table 5–3 • Isotypes (Classes) of Immunoglobulins*

Isotype	Heavy (H) chain
IgG	γ
IgA	α
IgM	μ
IgD	δ
IgE	ε

*In order of decreasing concentration

constant regions; the variable regions of both the light and heavy chains determine the antigenic specificity of the immunoglobulin. Each immunoglobulin contains two identical antigen-combining sites. The term **idiotype** refers to the antigen-binding site of the immunoglobulin molecule. The idiotype is composed of the variable regions of both the heavy and light chains and is unique for each antibody.

Types and Functions of Immunoglobulin Isotypes

IgG is the predominant immunoglobulin (Table 5–4). It is present in both the vascular and extravascular spaces. Further separation of IgG reveals four distinct subclasses, designated IgG1, IgG2, IgG3, and IgG4. Each subclass has different properties. For example, IgG1 and IgG3 are effective in activating complement via the classic pathway. In contrast, IgG2 is only minimally active, and IgG4 cannot activate these mediators of inflammation. IgG1 and IgG3 primarily react against protein antigens, whereas IgG2 and IgG4 react against polysaccharide antigens such as those associated with the capsules of pneumococci and Haemophilus influenzae.

Although **IgA** is the immunoglobulin in the second highest concentration in the serum, its major physiologic role appears to be in external secretions. IgA predominates in lachrymal, nasopharyngeal, salivary, respiratory, and gastrointestinal fluids. Plasma cells located in the submucosa of these organs synthesize and secrete this immunoglobulin, which is then linked to a small protein produced by the epithelial cells, called secretory piece. The IgA-secretory piece complex is secreted externally. Secretory IgA is important in local protection against tissue invasion by many pathogens. The role of serum IgA is conjectural; it is not a precursor of the secretory form.

The largest immunoglobulin is **IgM**, with a molecular weight of approximately 900,000. Structurally, this immunoglobulin is composed of five subunits, each consisting of two μ heavy chains and two light chains. IgM usually is the first detectable antibody synthesized following antigenic challenge. A sensitive relationship exists between the circulating levels of IgG and IgM antibodies. Specific IgM antibodies facilitate the production of antigen-specific IgG. In turn, this IgG inhibits the further production of IgM. The levels of IgG antibodies generally rise to higher concentrations and persist appreciably longer than the levels of the IgM class.

The two other classes of immunoglobulins are minor serum components. The function of serum **IgD** is unknown, but this

Table 5–4 • Properties of Immunoglobulins

Property	IgG	IgA	IgM	IgD	IgE
Serum concentration (mg/mL)	12.4	2.5	1.2	0.03	0.0003
Molecular weight	160,000	170,000; 385,000*	900,000	180,000	200,000
Sedimentation coefficient	7S	7S (9S, 11S, 13S)	19S	7S	8S
Biologic half-life (days)†	23	6	5	2.8	2.4
Synthesis rate (mg/kg/day)	34	24	3.3	0.4	0.0023
Percent intravascular	45	42	80	75	51
Biologic function	Principal serum antibody	Secretory antibody	Initial response to antigen	Unknown	Anaphylactic reaction

*The molecular weight of serum IgA is 170,000. Secretory IgA consists of two units of IgA combined with "secretory piece" (MW 385,000).
†The biological half-life of IgG is a function of serum concentration: t½ is prolonged with low levels, shortened with high concentrations. The half-lives of other immunoglobulins are independent of serum concentrations.

93

antibody does appear to be an important antigen receptor on a subset of B lymphocytes. **IgE** is responsible for allergic reactions. This immunoglobulin is able to bind and remain fixed to basophils and tissue mast cells; a reaction between tissue-bound IgE and the appropriate antigen (allergen) induces the release from basophils of histamine and other mediators of the allergic response. IgE may play an essential role in initiating inflammatory reactions.

Analysis of Serum Proteins

Serum protein electrophoresis is the major clinical tool for detecting immunoglobulin abnormalities. This method of separation is based on the net electrical charge of serum proteins. Most immunoglobulins reside in the gamma-globulin region, the slowest anodal migrating fraction. Thus, the term **gamma globulins** has been used synonymously with **immunoglobulins**. The two are not identical, however. Some antibodies migrate more rapidly and are found in the beta or the $alpha_2$ regions of the electrophoretic pattern.

Three types of immunoglobulin alterations can be identified by serum electrophoresis (Figure 5–11):

1. **Hypogammaglobulinemia**: a reduction in the total quantity of immunoglobulins
2. **Polyclonal gammopathy**: a diffuse or heterogeneous increase in many antibody species
3. **Monoclonal gammopathy**: the presence of an excess amount of a single, homogenous immunoglobulin.

The immunoglobulin in monoclonal gammopathy consists of only a single type of light chain and a single type of heavy chain. Furthermore, it has specificity for only a single antigen. Monoclonal proteins are characteristically seen in diseases such as multiple myeloma and macroglobulinemia (see Chapter 6). On an electrophoretic tracing, the single protein species appears as a tall, narrow-based spike. In contrast, polyclonal gammopathies produce a broad-based, rounded, and irregular increase in gamma globulins. This type of abnormality is seen in many chronic infections and diffuse inflammatory diseases. Polyclonal gammopathies are a mixture of different antibodies. They contain both kappa and lambda light chains and different types of heavy chains.

Although serum electrophoresis provides a useful screening procedure, it has limitations. It does not distinguish between the

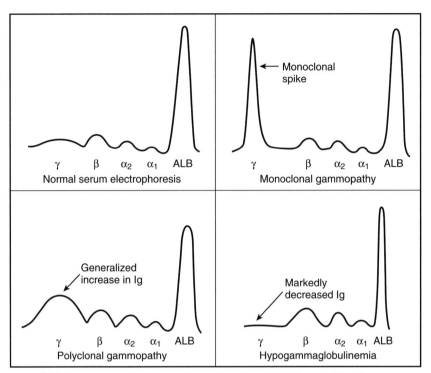

Figure 5–11. Serum protein electrophoretic patterns. As discussed in the text, a monoclonal "spike" represents the overproduction of a single species of antibody. A polyclonal pattern occurs when there is excessive production of multiple antibodies. ALB = albumin.

different immunoglobulin isotypes. Serum electrophoresis cannot identify a monoclonal gammopathy as an IgG, IgA, or IgM abnormality. Also, it may not be able to detect a deficiency in one type of immunoglobulin if the levels of others are normal or increased. For example, because IgA constitutes only a minor fraction of the total immunoglobulins, a patient with an IgA deficiency has a normal electrophoretic pattern. More specific determinations require additional testing. **Immunoelectrophoresis** and **immunofixation** are sensitive techniques for identifying qualitative abnormalities, and low levels of various immunoglobulin isotypes can be measured quantitatively.

Chapter

6 Lymphocyte and Immune Disorders

Lymphopenia and Lymphocytosis

In normal individuals the blood lymphocyte count ranges from 1500 to 4000 cells/μL. **Lymphopenia**, a decrease in the number of circulating lymphocytes, can be seen in several pathologic processes (Table 6–1). Apparently normal individuals may also have a modest reduction in the number of these cells for unidentified reasons. This finding by itself is not a cause of concern.

Infectious diseases, neoplasms, and connective-tissue syndromes can all be associated with lymphopenia. Probably the most common cause of a pathological lymphopenia at present is the acquired immune deficiency syndrome (AIDS). In this disorder progressive depletion of T lymphocytes occurs.

Transient reductions in blood lymphocytes routinely occur in the acute phases of many bacterial and viral infections. For example, the initial phases of pneumococcal pneumonia may be associated with a transient but marked reduction in blood lymphocyte counts. Lymphopenia may occur in certain chronic infections such as tuberculosis. It has also been observed in patients with disseminated neoplasms. In some of these patients it is correlated with a poor prognosis. Reduced blood lymphocyte counts are also observed in patients with diffuse connective-tissue diseases, particularly systemic lupus erythematosus (SLE). In these patients the reduction may be caused by antilymphocytic antibodies, which can cause either an autoimmune destruction of lymphoid cells or a redistribution between the tissue reserves and the blood compartment.

Lymphopenia may also result from therapy for various diseases. Cytotoxic drugs and irradiation cause lymphopenia. Irradiation-induced lymphopenia can be prolonged. In animals such as mice, rats, and rabbits steroids cause rapid lympholysis, but in

Table 6–1 • Causes of Lymphopenia and Lymphocytosis

Lymphopenia (<1500/cu mm)
- No apparent disease
- Acute inflammatory disorders
- Corticosteroids
- Immune deficiency diseases
- Chronic infections
- Neoplasms
- Connective-tissue diseases

Lymphocytosis (>4000/cu mm)
- Infectious mononucleosis and related diseases
- Pertussis (whooping cough)
- Lymphoid malignancies
  - Chronic lymphocytic leukemia
  - Leukemic phase of lymphomas
  - Acute lymphoblastic leukemia

humans they are not primarily lympholytic. Rather, they cause an abrupt decrease in the number of blood lymphocytes because of sequestration of these cells into lymphoid tissues and the bone marrow. Steroid effects are maximal 4 to 6 hours after a single intravenous injection of hydrocortisone. In 24 hours the blood lymphocyte count returns to normal.

In contrast to lymphopenia, **lymphocytosis** is rarely encountered in normal adults. The most common causes of blood lymphocyte counts in excess of 4000 cells/μL are specific viral infections, such as infectious mononucleosis, and neoplasms of the lymphoid system. In mononucleosis, many of the circulating lymphocytes have an atypical morphologic appearance. They are larger than the typical small lymphocyte that predominates in normal blood. These atypical cells have a basophilic cytoplasm, often with vacuoles. The nuclear chromatin is less dense and may show prominent nucleoli. The shape of the nucleus is often irregular. These cells have been identified as transformed T lymphocytes that are responding to B lymphocytes infected with the causative agent, the Epstein-Barr virus (EBV). The virus itself does not usually infect T cells; its tropism is limited to B lymphocytes and certain nasopharyngeal cells.

An increase in blood lymphocytes with morphologic changes similar to those found in infectious mononucleosis can also be seen in other infectious diseases, such as those caused by cytomegalovirus (CMV), viral hepatitis, toxoplasmosis, and in the early stages of HIV infection. In these diseases, the total lymphocyte count is often normal or only slightly increased. In young children, one infectious disease, pertussis (whooping cough), is associated with a markedly elevated lymphocyte count. Unlike mononucleosis, the lymphocytes seen on blood smears of patients with pertussis are small, normal-appearing cells. This infectious process appears to transiently mobilize lymphocytes from lymphatic tissues into the blood.

Lymphocytosis is also seen in neoplasms affecting the lymphoid system. Chronic lymphocytic leukemia (CLL), the most common type of leukemia seen in the United States, is characterized by persistent elevations of the blood lymphocyte count. Most of the circulating cells appear to be small, mononuclear cells, which are morphologically indistinguishable from normal lymphocytes. As will be discussed, more than 95% of patients with CLL have a clonal B cell neoplasm. The other 5% have uncommon forms of lymphoid leukemias including malignancies affecting T or B cells. Lymphoblasts (the immature precursor cells) are the characteristic cells present in the circulation of patients with acute lymphoblastic leukemia.

Histocompatibility

Major histocompatibility complex (MHC) molecules are expressed on all nucleated cells and in humans are referred to as **human leukocyte antigens (HLA).** The genes that encode the MHC antigens are clustered together in the MHC region found on the short arm of chromosome 6 (Figure 6–1). HLA molecules, together with T-cell receptors (TCR), play a critical role in the immune response as well as in the general process by which an individual discriminates at the molecular and cellular level between self and nonself or foreign antigens. The first step in an immune response is the binding of a processed antigenic peptide to an HLA molecule, followed by interaction of a T-cell receptor with the HLA/peptide complex. The formation of such a complex leads to T-cell activation. There are two types of structurally similar HLA molecules, referred to as class I and class II molecules. The class I molecules, HLA-A, HLA-B, and HLA-C, interact with TCR on $CD8^+$ T cells. The class II molecules, HLA-DR, HLA-DQ, and HLA-DP, interact with TCR on $CD4^+$ T cells.

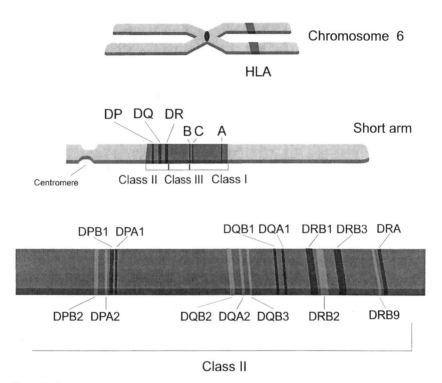

Figure 6–1. Genetic map of the human major histocompatibility complex on chromosome 6.

HLA class I molecules are heterodimers consisting of a highly polymorphic heavy chain and a nonpolymorphic light chain (β_2 microglobulin) encoded on chromosome 15. The heavy-chain amino acids fold into three distinct regions, α-1, α-2, and α-3. All of the polymorphic amino acid residues are found in the α-1 and α-2 domains, which are known from crystallographic analysis to constitute the **peptide binding groove** formed by a platform of β-pleated sheets overlain by two α-helical structures (Figure 6–2).

Unlike class I molecules, which are expressed on all nucleated cells, HLA class II molecules are normally expressed only on B lymphocytes, monocytes, dendritic cells, Langerhans cells, and some endothelial cells. They are also present on activated T cells and on immature myeloid cells (blasts). HLA class II molecules are heterodimers consisting of a highly polymorphic β chain and an α chain. In HLA-DR molecules the α chain is invariant, whereas in the HLA-DQ molecules both the α chain and the β chain are polymorphic. The amino-terminal domains of class II α and β chains are

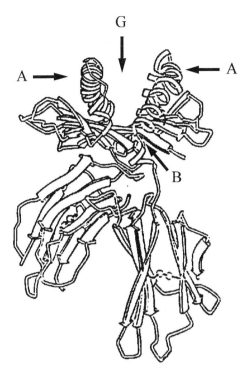

G

A →   ← A

B

Figure 6–2. Schematic of an HLA molecule. The arrows labeled "A" point out the α helices, the arrow labeled "B" points out the antiparallel β strands, and the arrow labeled "G" points out the peptide binding groove. Adapted from Stern, L.J., & Wiley, D.C. (1994). Antigenic peptide binding by Class I and Class II histocompatibility proteins. Structure, 2, 245–251.

folded into a platform of eight antiparallel β strands topped by two α helices, forming a structure very similar to that of HLA class I molecules. The large groove formed between the α helices in both class I and class II molecules provides a single site for binding an antigenic peptide. The charge and size of the side chains of polymorphic amino acids that line the peptide binding groove produce subtle conformational and charge differences among HLA allelic products. In fact, within the peptide binding groove of an HLA molecule several smaller cavities or "pockets" can be identified that can accommodate the side chains of a bound peptide (Figure 6–3). The distinctive binding site of each molecule may explain the apparent preferential binding of sets of specific antigenic peptides to particular HLA molecules. Characteristic peptide binding motifs have been identified for HLA molecules. Preferential binding of certain antigenic peptides to some HLA class II alleles and not to others may explain, at least partly, the association of certain diseases involving an immune response with particular HLA haplotypes.

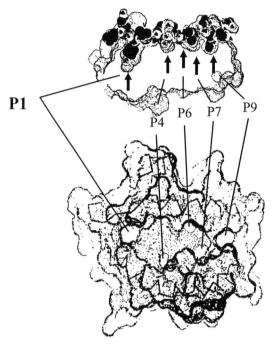

Figure 6–3. Schematic of the pockets in an HLA class II binding groove. The upper figure represents a side view of the binding groove with a bound peptide. The arrows point out the side chain pockets. The lower figure shows the top view of the molecular surface of the binding groove. Adapted from Stern, L.J., Brown, J.H., Jardetzky, T.S., et al. (1994). Crystal structure of the human class II MHC protein HLA-DR1 complexed with an influenza virus peptide. Nature, 368, 215–221, p. 220.

Immune Deficiency Syndromes

Disorders characterized by reduced ability to mount immune responses are subdivided into two groups: (1) those in which there is no underlying disorder **(primary immune deficiency disorders)**, and (2) those associated with a causative pathologic process **(secondary immune deficiency states)**. Within each category, defects may be classified according to the major pathophysiologic manifestations: failure of humoral antibody formation (hypogammaglobulinemia), deficient cell-mediated immunity, or combined failures of both defense mechanisms.

Primary Immune Deficiency Disorders

The division of peripheral lymphocytes into two populations, each responsible for a different type of immunity, lends itself to a model

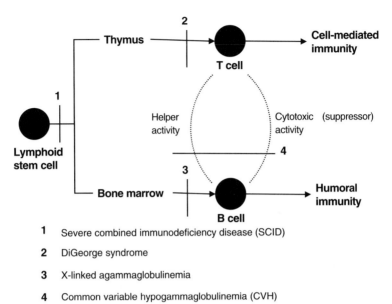

1 Severe combined immunodeficiency disease (SCID)

2 DiGeorge syndrome

3 X-linked agammaglobulinemia

4 Common variable hypogammaglobulinemia (CVH)

Figure 6–4. Several congenital and inherited immunodeficiency syndromes can be viewed as cellular blocks in the normal maturation sequence of lymphocytes.

encompassing many immune deficiencies (Figure 6–4). Abnormalities can affect the common lymphocyte stem cell, causing defects in both cell-mediated and humoral immunity, or be limited to defects in either T or B cells. A brief description of sentinel disorders follows.

Severe Combined Immunodeficiencies

Severe combined immunodeficiencies (SCID) are a group of inherited disorders in which both cell-mediated and humoral immunity are markedly impaired. Thus they represent the most severe immunologic failure. The syndrome is inheritable as an autosomal recessive trait or as an X-linked trait resulting from a deficiency in the production of the gamma chain of the IL-2 receptor. The binding of IL-2 by this receptor permits the clonal expansion of stimulated T cells. The IL-2 receptor consists of three polypeptide chains, alpha, beta, and gamma. The gamma chain also is a component of the receptors for other interleukins, including IL-4, IL-7, IL-11, and IL-15. Early lymphoid precursors in this disease appear to lack functional receptors for all of these interleukins and thus are unable to either proliferate or mature into immunologically functional cells.

One of the identified causes of the autosomal form of SCID is a deficiency in the lymphocyte enzyme adenosine deaminase (ADA). This enzyme is required to prevent the toxic accumulation of the metabolite deoxyinosine in lymphocytes. Excess deoxyinosine is converted to deoxyadenosine triphosphate (dATP), which inhibits the DNA repair reactions in lymphocytes and ultimately results in their apoptotic death. An uncommon form of SCID can result from a deficiency in another intracellular enzyme, nucleoside phosphorylase.

Although SCID has several genetic causes, all manifest a common phenotype. Clinical manifestations appear within the first 3 months of life and include recurrent infections (frequently with organisms of low pathogenicity), severe diarrhea, chronic skin rashes, a failure to thrive, and death, generally within the first year of life. Some of the clinical manifestations may be due to graft-versus-host disease resulting from the transplacental passage of maternal lymphocytes that react against parenterally derived antigens.

As would be expected from the nature of the defect, laboratory studies indicate a marked reduction in T lymphocytes. In some patients B cells may be present, but they appear to be functionally impaired. Other patients lack B cells entirely. Additional abnormalities in children with SCID include profound hypogammaglobulinemia and the absence of cell-mediated and humoral responses to test antigens. Immunologic reconstitution has been achieved with bone marrow transplants and, in the case of ADA deficiency, partial reconstruction with the administration of the enzyme linked to a carrier molecule (polyethylene glycol [PEG-ADA]). Immune function in ADA-deficient children has been established using gene therapy, that is, by inserting the ADA gene in either the patient's lymphocytes or the patient's bone marrow stem cells.

Defective MHC Expression ("Bare Lymphocyte Syndrome")

Another group of immune deficiencies results from failure of accessory cells to express either MHC class I or class II antigens. These molecules are essential for presenting antigens to T cells. Class I antigens, which are expressed on all nucleated cells and platelets, are required for binding of the antigen-presenting cell to CD8+ T cells. Class II molecules are constitutively expressed on monocytes, B lymphocytes, dendritic cells, and thymic epithelial cells. They are also present on activated (but not resting) T cells. These molecules function in antigen presentation to CD4+ cells.

An autosomal recessive disorder characterized by a deficiency in the expression of class II MHC antigens has been recently described. Because of a failure of gene transcription, the formation of these molecules is markedly reduced, resulting in a severe immunodeficiency. Affected children have severe and protracted diarrhea and recurrent infections, primarily of the upper and lower airways. The syndrome is fatal during the first or second decade of life. The laboratory abnormalities are predictable; these children have markedly reduced numbers of CD4$^+$ cells but normal numbers of both CD8$^+$ T cells and B cells. Because of the lack of T-cell help, there is profound hypogammaglobulinemia. Class I MHC deficiencies have also been reported, but are extremely uncommon; they too result in a combined-system immune deficiency.

Congenital Thymic Aplasia (DiGeorge Syndrome)

Congenital thymic aplasia (DiGeorge syndrome) is caused by a failure of embryological development of the third and fourth pharyngeal pouches, which causes a congenital absence or hypoplasia of both the thymus and the parathyroid glands. This abnormality causes both severe hypoparathyroidism with hypocalcemic tetany and a profound immune deficiency, primarily involving the cell-mediated immune system. Affected children often have many other abnormalities including abnormal facies and congenital heart defects. The immunologic defect manifests itself early in life, usually within the first few months after birth. These children suffer from recurrent or chronic infections with various viral, bacterial, fungal, and protozoal organisms. Immunologically, they have a profound lymphopenia as a result of failure of T-cell lymphopoiesis. B lymphocytes are present but humoral immune responses are variably depressed because of a lack of T-cell help. This syndrome, if not treated, is fatal during the first year of life. Some patients with this syndrome have been successfully treated with fetal thymus transplants.

X-linked Agammaglobulinemia (Bruton's Agammaglobulinemia)

X-linked agammaglobulinemia (Bruton's agammaglobulinemia) is an X-linked disorder that is the prototype of a pure B-cell deficiency. Characteristically, boys with this disorder develop recurrent respiratory and skin infections, primarily caused by extracellular pyogenic bacteria (pneumococci, *Haemophilus influenzae*). In contrast, children with agammaglobulinemia respond to most viral infections in a manner similar to that seen in normal individuals. Laboratory data include a normal number of total circulating lymphocytes but a profound absence of B cells. Either immunoglobulin is absent or immunoglobin levels are markedly depressed, and humoral immune responses to test antigens are absent. In contrast, cell-mediated immune responses are normal.

Recent studies have defined the genetic defect. X-linked agammaglobulinemia is caused by a mutation mapped to the long arm of the X chromosome, which codes for a cytoplasmic tyrosine kinase. This specific mutation has been designated **btk** (Bruton's tyrosine kinase). It is known that this gene is expressed in early B-cell development and serves a vital, but as yet undefined, role in B-cell maturation. The genetic defect can be detected in female carriers. Children with this defect can survive into adult life with appropriate treatment (antibiotics and replacement gammaglobulin).

Hyper-IgM Syndrome

Hyper-IgM syndrome is characterized by elevated concentrations of serum IgM associated with an absence of IgA and IgE and extremely low levels of IgG. In about 70% of cases this syndrome is inherited as an X-linked recessive trait. The clinical manifestations closely resemble those seen in X-linked agammaglobulinemia. Patients with this disorder experience recurrent pyogenic infections. In addition to the humoral immune deficiencies, many patients develop autoantibodies against the formed elements of the blood, which commonly causes severe and prolonged neutropenia.

Immunologic studies have revealed important information about the cause of this abnormality, especially emphasizing the importance of physical contact between T and B lymphocytes. Immunoglobulin class switching requires the interaction of T lymphocytes with the antigen-stimulated B cell, resulting in B-cell heavy chain isotype switching, from IgM to IgG, IgA, or IgE, depending upon the type of T lymphocyte binding (T helper 1 or T helper 2). This interaction requires the binding of CD40, an antigen located on B cells, with its ligand (CD40L) expressed on activated T cells. The ligand is coded for by a gene present on the long arm of the X chromosome. This interaction is also responsible for generating B memory cells and for the formation of germinal centers in lymphoid organs, so biopsies of lymph nodes of patient with the hyper-IgM syndrome show a lack of germinal centers.

Common Variable Hypogammaglobulinemia (CVH)

Common variable hypogammaglobulinemia (CVH) is a heterogeneous syndrome consisting of several disorders, all characterized by reduced levels of immunoglobulins. The hypogammaglobulinemia appears after a period of apparently normal immunoglobulin production. The age of onset varies from early infancy to late adult life, but most commonly is in the second or third decade. Both sexes are affected equally. The clinical manifestations are highly variable and partly reflect the severity of the immunodeficiency. Patients with severely reduced levels of immunoglobulins are susceptible to infections caused by encapsulated pyogenic bacteria. The respiratory tract tends to be the major target of these organisms. If untreated, these patients usually succumb to chronic respiratory failure or bronchiectasis. Cell-mediated immune responses are either normal or only minimally impaired and these patients are not highly susceptible to infections by intracellular organisms.

This syndrome has several peculiar aspects. Affected patients show a high incidence of both allergic and autoimmune disorders. The autoimmune complications include antibody-mediated destruction of red cells, platelets, or neutrophils. It appears that in certain patients, the humoral immune system is unable to recognize external pathogenic organisms as foreign, but can mount antibody responses against the individual's own cells. Patients with CVH may show a generalized hyperplasia of lymphoid tissues. This can manifest itself as splenomegaly, lymphadenopathy, or a nodular hyperplasia of intestinal lymphoid tissue. The incidence of malignant lymphomas also is high in patients with CVH.

The pathogenesis of this syndrome (Figure 6–5) is highly variable. In 10% to 15% of affected patients there is a marked deficiency of B lymphocytes. In these patients, the abnormality appears to be phenotypically similar to Bruton's agammaglobulinemia. Most patients with CVH, however, have normal numbers of B lymphocytes in the blood and tissues, suggesting other pathogenic mechanisms. In some the immune defect appears to result from an intrinsic abnormality of B lymphocytes, which either are unable to proliferate in response to an antigenic challenge or have a block in their ability to terminally differentiate into plasma cells. In 5% to 10% of CVH patients, there is excessive T-suppressor-cell activity; isolated B cells, separated from autologous T cells, can normally

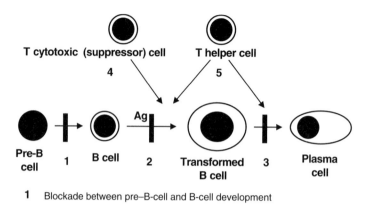

1 Blockade between pre–B-cell and B-cell development

2 Inability of B cell to transform and proliferate after antigenic stimulation

3 Inability of B cell to mature into plasma cells

4 Excessive T-cytotoxic–cell activity

5 Lack of T-helper–cell activity

Figure 6–5. Possible pathogenic mechanisms responsible for common variable hypogammaglobulinemia. Recent studies suggest that the most common defect may be a lack of T-cell help.

proliferate, mature, and differentiate into antibody-producing plasma cells. Conversely, the patient's T cells are able to inhibit the reactivity of normal B cells.

Recent studies suggest that the most common cause of this syndrome is defective T-cell help. Patients appear to have abnormalities in the release of B-cell stimulating factors by T lymphocytes. The exact factors missing in these patients have not been defined, but it is known that multiple interleukins function in the processes of B-cell activation, proliferation, and terminal differentiation into plasma cells. In a subset of these patients, the production of interleukins by T cells is normal but the patient's B cells are unable to respond to these growth factors.

Regardless of the pathogenic abnormality, treatment of CVH is primarily supportive, with replacement gammaglobulin and antibiotics for infections.

Selective Absence of IgA

Selective absence of IgA is the most common of the primary immunodeficiencies. It occurs in approximately 1 in 600 individuals. Patients with this disorder lack IgA in both the serum and external secretions. In contrast, IgG and IgM levels are usually normal. Despite the lack of IgA, which is thought to be important for immune protection at mucosal surfaces, most of these patients do not suffer from recurrent infections. Only a small percentage of those affected have an increased frequency of infections, and these occur primarily in the respiratory or gastrointestinal tract. One possible cause for these infections is a coexistent deficiency in one or more of the IgG subsets.

Most IgA-deficient subjects maintain mucosal immunity by externally secreting IgM or IgG. Patients lacking IgA show a higher than expected incidence of allergic and autoimmune disorders. These patients can have anti-IgA antibodies, the development of which may be associated with anaphylactic reaction to transfusion of blood or plasma. Lymphocyte studies indicate that almost all affected patients have IgA-bearing lymphocytes, suggesting that the defect in production of this immunoglobulin is caused by a maturation block in the differentiation of these cells into IgA-secreting plasma cells.

Secondary Immune Deficiency Disorders

Transient secondary immune deficiencies are common. They frequently occur during the course of many acute and chronic diseases and can be a major cause of increased morbidity and mortality. The increasing use of drugs capable of altering immune responsiveness is an additional cause of deficiency states.

In contrast to these conditions, which tend to be self-limited, there are persistent forms of secondary immune deficiencies. Two of the major causes are infection with the human immunodeficiency virus (HIV), leading to AIDS, and neoplasms affecting the lymphoid system.

Acquired Immune Deficiency Syndrome

AIDS is a syndrome resulting from infection with HIV. This retrovirus has the ability to enter, propagate in, and ultimately destroy CD4$^+$ T cells. The result is a progressive loss of these cells, severely crippling host defense mechanisms. CD4$^+$ T cells are essential in virtually all host defense mechanisms (Figure 6–6). Ultimately, the impairment in immune defenses renders the patient susceptible to infections by organisms that do not normally cause disease in healthy individuals **(opportunistic infections)** and certain forms of cancer (particularly a rare form of skin cancer, Kaposi's sarcoma, and non-Hodgkin's lymphoma).

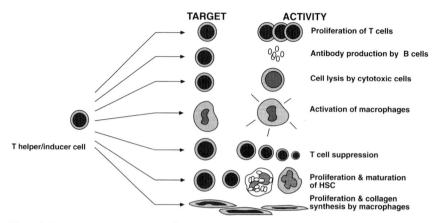

Figure 6–6. Multiple roles of CD4⁺ (helper/inducer) T cells in homeostasis. HSC = hematopoietic stem cell.

The first cases of AIDS were reported in 1980. Unfortunately, the disease has rapidly reached epidemic proportions; it is estimated that between 1 and 1.5 million Americans and more than 14 million people worldwide are infected with the virus. It is currently believed that all infected patients will ultimately develop AIDS. The interval between infection and the development of manifestations of AIDS (the latent period) tends to be long, averaging 10 years, but it can vary widely. Some patients develop AIDS within 2 to 3 years of infection, whereas another small group show no evidence of an immune deficiency after more than 12 years.

Although a comprehensive discussion of AIDS is beyond the scope of this manual, it is useful to review three aspects: the life cycle of the virus, the central role of CD4⁺ cells in the maintenance of the immune system, and the clinical features of the syndrome. The HIV retrovirus is an RNA virus. It consists of a protein envelope surrounding a core of RNA. The protein envelope has tropism; it binds specifically to the CD4 molecule. In conjunction with a newly described second receptor, a chemokine receptor, viral binding permits the viral core to enter the cytoplasm of CD4⁺ lymphocytes. One component of the viral core is the enzyme **reverse transcriptase**, which is capable of transcribing the genetic information contained in the viral RNA into DNA. (The term "reverse transcriptase" is applied because transcription is the reverse of the normal mechanism, in which DNA is transcribed into RNA.)

The newly formed DNA is then transported to the cell's nucleus, where it is integrated into the cell's own DNA. When the cell is activated, the viral-derived DNA is then transcribed into new RNA and subsequently into new proteins, resulting in the formation of a new virus. This is shed from the cell by a budding process and can infect additional CD4$^+$ cells. The life cycle of HIV is depicted in Figure 6–7. It should be noted that other cells, such as macrophages, also express small amounts of the CD4 antigen and are potential targets for infection.

In the process of viral shedding, the host cell is destroyed. Through mechanisms that are not well understood, the number of CD4$^+$ cells is progressively reduced. As with many other cellular systems, normal individuals have extensive reserves and thus do not experience the consequences of a deficiency until these cells are profoundly depleted. In uninfected individuals, the normal number of CD4$^+$ cells in the circulation is between 800 and 1500 cells/μL. Most patients with HIV infection do not show an increased susceptibility to infections until the CD4$^+$ cell count falls below 200 cells/μL. Figure 6–8 shows the temporal changes in CD4$^+$ cell counts in a patient with typical HIV infection.

The clinical course of HIV infection has been subdivided into several stages. At the time of infection, a minority of infected individuals develop an acute illness resembling infectious mononucleosis, characterized by fever, lymphadenopathy, and skin rashes. These manifestations generally last for 2 to 6 weeks before spontaneous resolution.

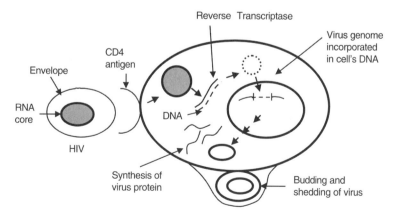

Figure 6–7. The life cycle of HIV. The virus itself is composed of an envelope protein, which can bind to the CD4 receptor, an RNA core, and the enzyme reverse transcriptase. Upon entering a cell, the reverse transcriptase transcribes the RNA into DNA, which is subsequently incorporated into the cell's own DNA.

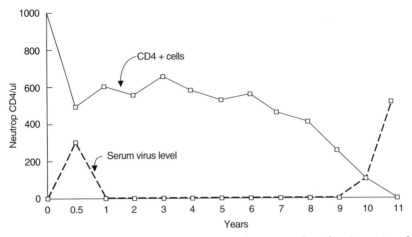

Figure 6–8. Typical changes in the CD4 counts of an HIV-infected patient. Note that the latent period, the interval between infection and the onset of symptoms, averages approximately 10 years.

During the first few weeks after infection, antibodies to the virus develop. These antibodies can be detected in routine testing for HIV infection. The average time interval between infection and the appearance of antibodies is 22 days, and it appears that nearly everyone who is infected with the virus will develop antibodies within 3 to 6 months.

In the typical infected patient, the initial infection is followed by an abrupt decrease in the number of CD4$^+$ cells to 500 to 600 cells/µL. This is followed by an asymptomatic (latent) period, during which the CD4 count tends to either remain relatively constant or decline at a slow rate. Ultimately, this plateau phase is followed by another rapid decrease in the CD4 count. Once the level falls below 200 cells/µL, reserves are depleted and the individual becomes susceptible to infections by organisms such as *Pneumocystis carinii, Toxoplasma gondii, Cytomegalovirus, Candida,* and *Mycobacterium tuberculosis* and *avium-intracellulare.* He or she also is at risk for developing Kaposi's sarcoma or lymphoma, two neoplasms that are probably of viral origin. Most patients survive 1 to 2 years after the onset of the first opportunistic infection or the development of a neoplasm. Therapy with multiple drugs, each aimed at inhibiting a selected phase of the viral life cycle, holds promise of both reducing morbidity and prolonging life span.

AIDS clearly demonstrates the pivotal role of CD4$^+$ cells in immune homeostasis (see Figure 6–6). These cells regulate the numbers and activities of most other host defense cells. For example, they release soluble mediators, which attract, localize, and activate macrophages and thus are essential for the killing of intracellular organisms. They also synthesize and secrete cytokines, which induce the proliferation, maturation, and differentiation of B cells. CD4 cells also activate cytotoxic T cells, which can kill both tumor and virally infected cells. In addition, the CD4 subset produces hematopoietic growth factors, important in promoting myeloid cell development, and interleukins, essential for the proliferative expansion of lymphocytes.

HIV is transmitted sexually, by contaminated blood, and neonatally from an infected mother to her fetus. Sexual transmission can occur through either heterosexual or homosexual contact. It is important to recognize that this virus is not spread by casual contact or by inhalation. Health-care workers can be infected by accidental exposure to blood or blood-containing fluids, so they must be especially vigilant in adhering to the Universal Precaution safeguards.

Neoplasms Affecting the Lymphoid System

Neoplastic tumors of the B lymphocyte system can be considered clonal proliferations of B cells arrested at a specific stage in the normal maturation sequence. The term **arrest** implies that the cells can progress to a specific maturation stage but are blocked in their terminal differentiation. **Clonality** indicates that all of the tumor cells are derived from a single precursor. As a result, all daughter cells display identical features. In the case of B cells, this implies that all have the same immunoglobulin gene rearrangements, resulting in the elaboration of a single antibody with specificity for one antigenic determinant.

Table 6–2 shows an overview of the normal maturation of B cells and some of the malignant counterparts representing arrests at each stage of development. Most cases of acute lymphoblastic leukemia result from the neoplastic transformation of a clone of cells arrested at the pre-B-cell stage. Malignancies affecting small resting B lymphocytes include both chronic lymphocytic leukemia (CLL) and low-grade forms of non-Hodgkin's lymphoma (NHL). Several different malignancies can be considered counterparts of antigen-stimulated B cells, including the more aggressive forms of NHL and Waldenstrom's macroglobulinemia. The neoplastic equivalent of the plasma cell is multiple myeloma. One of the common characteristics seen in many of these B-cell malignancies is a pro-

Table 6–2 • B-Cell Malignancies Resulting from Arrests in the Normal Maturation Sequence

Stages of Normal Maturation	Pre-B cell	B cell	Activated B cell	Plasma cell
Malignancy	Acute lymphoblastic leukemia (ALL)	Chronic lymphocytic leukemia (CLL)	Macroglobulinemia	Multiple myeloma
			Hairy cell leukemia	
		Non-Hodgkin's lymphoma (low-grade)	Non-Hodgkin's lymphoma (intermediate- and high-grade)	
Immune Abnormality	None	Hypogammaglobulinemia	Monoclonal IgM	Monoclonal Ig and/or light chain

Ig = Immunoglobulin.

nounced impairment in the production of antibodies to environmental antigens, resulting in increased susceptibility to infection.

B-cell neoplasms are clonal diseases; thus all cells belonging to the clone express the same membrane-associated immunoglobulin. This criterion is often used to distinguish between a benign polyclonal proliferation of lymphocytes and a clonal neoplasm. In practice, the most convenient method for detecting clonality is to determine the type of light chain present on the cell membrane. In a normal individual or one with a nonclonal lymphoproliferative disorder, about half of the B cells express κ light chains and the other half Λ light chains. In a lymphomatous infiltrate, on the other hand, all the cells express the same kind of light chain, either κ or Λ.

Chronic Lymphocytic Leukemia
Chronic lymphocytic leukemia (CLL) is a malignancy characterized by the clonal proliferation and accumulation of immuno-

logically incompetent B lymphocytes. It is the commonest form of leukemia in the United States. CLL is generally a disease of the elderly, usually occurring in the sixth through the eighth decade of life. The primary diagnostic criterion is a persistent increase in the number of morphologically normal lymphocytes in the blood. In many patients, the total number of blood lymphocytes exceeds 100,000/μL. Despite these high counts, affected patients may be entirely asymptomatic; the disease is often accidentally discovered on routine examination.

One of the major characteristics of this disease is the slow accumulation of neoplastic cells. The median survival of affected patients is 5 to 7 years, and many patients live with the disease for more than 15 years. As the disease progresses, the number of neoplastic cells in lymphatic tissues usually increases gradually. This increase may manifest itself as lymphadenopathy, splenomegaly, and ultimately bone marrow failure caused by the marrow being replaced with neoplastic cells. Marrow replacement can result in an aregenerative anemia or thrombocytopenia.

CLL patients almost invariably have prominent defects in their humoral immune system. These can be summarized as follows:

- **Reduced antibody production** occurs in almost all patients. It can be demonstrated by subnormal or absent antibody responses to most vaccines.
- **Deficiencies in one or more immunoglobulin isotypes** can be found in 70% to 90% of affected patients.
- About 50% of affected patients, especially those with advanced disease, have a **panhypogammaglobulinemia** (a reduction in all immunoglobulins).
- The reduction in gamma globulin can be correlated with an **increased susceptibility to infections caused by encapsulated pyogenic organisms**. Patients with markedly impaired antibody production are particularly susceptible to infections with organisms such as pneumococci and *Hemophilus influenzae*.
- In contrast, **cell-mediated immunity is not markedly impaired** in the absence of immunosuppressive therapy.

In addition to this acquired immune deficiency, some patients develop **autoimmune phenomena**, most often autoimmune reactions directed against the formed elements of the blood (erythrocytes, platelets, neutrophils). In most patients, the autoantibodies apparently are not synthesized and secreted by the malignant cells.

This is suggested by the fact that the immunoglobulin isotype produced by the neoplasm is restricted to either a monoclonal IgM or a monoclonal IgM+IgD, whereas the autoreactive antibodies to red cells or platelets are polyclonal, generally IgG.

Typically, the neoplastic B cells in CLL express pan–B-cell antigens CD19 and CD20. Because the cells are monoclonal, all of the malignant lymphocytes will show the same membrane-associated immunoglobulin.

CLL cells also react with a single anti–T-cell antibody, CD5, leading to speculation about whether a normal population of $CD5^+$ B cells exists, and if so, about their function. Research has shown that $CD5^+$ B cells comprise a minor lymphoid subset in normal adults, about 10% of the circulating B-cell pool. In fetal life and newborn infants, on the other hand, $CD5^+$ B cells predominate. They also make up the majority of circulating B cells immediately after allogeneic bone marrow transplantation. Both the neonatal and the post-transplant periods are characterized by defective antibody production, an immune deficiency similar to that occurring in patients with CLL. Increased numbers of $CD5^+$ B cells also have been observed in patients with certain connective tissue diseases, such as rheumatoid arthritis and Sjögren's syndrome; both disorders are considered to be of autoimmune origin and, like CLL, are characterized by the elaboration of autoantibodies.

Based on these data, it has been postulated that $CD5^+$ B cells function as immune regulators. According to this thesis, the $CD5^+$ B cells in CLL may inhibit the functions of normal $CD5^-$ B cells, which produce antibodies directed at external antigens. Thus the $CD5^+$ B cells cause immune deficiency. Concomitantly, these cells augment the responses of self-reactive B cells capable of producing autoantibodies, causing autoimmunity.

Treatment of CLL is controversial. There is no evidence that therapy alters the survival of asymptomatic individuals. For those with symptomatic disease, palliation can be achieved with single-agent chemotherapy, combined cytotoxic drug regimens, or a new group of agents, the nucleoside analogs, which act by circumventing the enzyme adenosine deaminase.

Multiple Myeloma

Multiple myeloma is a clonal neoplasm of terminally differentiated plasma cells; these cells elaborate a homogenous immunoglobulin, a single type of free light chain, or both. Myeloma, like CLL, is a disease primarily of the elderly. It is characterized by two major features:

1. Infiltration of the bone marrow by an abnormal number of plasma cells. Morphologically, these cells may appear as typical plasma cells or have atypical or immature features.
2. The presence of a monoclonal protein in serum or urine. This can be identified as a monoclonal spike on serum or urine electrophoresis.

Some investigators include a third criterion, characteristic "punched-out" bone lesions. Although these are almost pathognomonic for myeloma, they are seen in only a few patients.

Although the malignant cell in myeloma is a plasma cell, idiotypic identification of myeloma proteins indicates that the same determinant can be found in cells as early in their maturation sequence as the pre-B-lymphocyte stage. This finding suggests that the neoplastic transformation may actually occur in an early cell committed to the B-cell lineage. This cell retains its capacity to proliferate and differentiate but is not controlled by normal regulatory mechanisms.

Depending on the relative quantities of light and heavy chains synthesized by the malignant clone of plasma cells, the monoclonal protein abnormality may lead to the formation of a complete immunoglobulin molecule, only the light chain portion of the molecule, or both a complete immunoglobulin molecule and free light chains. The light and heavy chains are synthesized on separate polyribosomes, and the production of heavy chains is the rate-limiting step.

A complete immunoglobulin molecule is large enough that it is not filtered at the renal glomerulus, so these antibodies are retained in the serum and can be identified as a monoclonal protein. In contrast, free light chains are small molecules that are completely cleared by glomerular filtration, so they are found only in the urine, not in the serum. Myeloma patients who synthesize only monoclonal light chains show a monoclonal protein in their urine, not in their serum. Myeloma plasma cells that have a disproportionate synthesis of light and heavy chains show both monoclonal spikes in the serum (the complete immunoglobulin molecule, composed of both the heavy and the light chains, forming a single protein spike) and in the urine (a monoclonal light chain). Thus, three distinct types of protein abnormalities can be recognized in patients with myeloma. These are summarized in Table 6–3.

Table 6–3 • Protein Abnormalities in Multiple Myeloma

Comparative Synthesis of Heavy and Light Chains	Monoclonal Abnormalities	
	Serum	Urine
H = L	+	0
H < L	+	+
L only	0	+

For any single patient, the quantity of the monoclonal protein is directly proportional to the total number of malignant cells. Thus, serial measurements of the monoclonal protein are the most accurate means of assessing progression of the disease or its response to therapy. In general, a 50% change in the concentration is considered significant. The serum level of β_2 microglobulin has also proven to be a useful prognostic indicator. Survival of patients with normal concentrations is appreciably longer than that of patients with elevated values. Recent studies have shown that the interleukin IL-6 may have an important pathogenic role as the major stimulus for the growth of malignant plasmablasts. Clinically, serum levels of IL-6 have implications for prognosis and monitoring.

Although patients with myeloma produce excessive quantities of a single immunoglobulin or light chain, their production of normal polyclonal antibodies is markedly impaired. As a result, they display a spectrum of increased susceptibility to infection similar to that of CLL patients. Although several mechanisms for the decrease in antibody production have been postulated, the cause is not known.

Myeloma has several concomitant clinical features. Patients with this disease often experience bone marrow failure as a result of the infiltration of plasma cells, which replace normal hematopoietic elements. A major complication of myeloma is renal failure, which is the cause of death in approximately one-third of affected patients. The renal failure is principally caused by the presence of free light chains in the renal tubules. In some patients, a certain type of monoclonal light chain seems to be partially reabsorbed by renal tubular cells, but the epithelial cells are unable to degrade these immunoglobulin fragments. Tubular fibrosis, tubular cell death, and renal failure are the ultimate results. The presence of light chains in the urine does not necessarily indicate that the patient will develop renal failure, however. Why some patients handle light chains without problems while others develop severe renal failure is not known. In some cases a light-chain derivative known as amyloid also is deposited in many tissues and organs, compromising function (see pages 120–122).

Another problem in patients with myeloma is excessive bone destruction. The plasma cells can release a soluble factor, osteoclast-activating factor (OAF), which mobilizes and activates osteoclasts, causing bone reabsorption. The resulting severe demineralization can lead to both pathologic fractures and intense bone pain. In addition, the calcium mobilized from the bone stores can lead to hypercalcemia and hypercalcinuria. The "punched-out" bone lesions already described are seen on x-ray as holes in the bone. They differ from the osteolytic lesions seen with other neoplastic diseases in that they are not surrounded by a sclerotic zone of new bone formation.

Patients with myeloma typically survive for 2 to 3 years. Some patients have a rapidly progressive disease and die within a few months of diagnosis, whereas others have "smoldering" disease and may live for several years. Treatment at present is palliative; it can increase survival time but is not curative.

Macroglobulinemia

Macroglobulinemia is a lymphoid malignancy characterized by excessive production of a monoclonal IgM immunoglobulin. The neoplastic cells have features of both lymphocytes and plasma cells. They are frequently referred to as **lymphocytoid plasma cells** or **plasmacytoid lymphocytes**. Immunologically, they resemble a transitional cell arrested at a stage intermediate between a lymphocyte and a plasma cell. Like lymphocytes, they show surface immunoglobulins, but like plasma cells, they have high concentrations of cytoplasmic immunoglobulins. Clinically, many patients with macroglobulinemia appear to have a disease resembling CLL or a low-grade non-Hodgkin's lymphoma. They may show lymphocytosis, lymphadenopathy, hepatosplenomegaly, and bone marrow infiltration. Unlike myeloma, macroglobulinemia is not a bone-destroying disease. Patients with this condition do not usually develop bone lesions, renal failure, or hypercalcemia.

One of the major problems in patients with macroglobuline-mia results from the presence of large quantities of the high–

molecular-weight IgM in the serum. This can impede blood flow, a condition known as the **hyperviscosity syndrome**. Manifestations are caused by decreased blood flow to vital organs, especially the central nervous system (with results ranging from mild headaches or focal neurologic defects to coma and convulsions), the cardiopulmonary system (primarily congestive heart failure), and the eyes. A bleeding diathesis may also be seen. Because most IgM is an intravascular protein, transient improvement in the hyperviscosity syndrome can be rapidly achieved with plasmapheresis.

Monoclonal Gammopathies of Undetermined Significance

In the course of routinely evaluating patients, a monoclonal serum protein may be discovered as an incidental finding. Most patients with this finding are elderly and, despite careful evaluation, show no evidence of a B-cell malignancy. In many of these individuals, the concentration of the monoclonal protein remains stable for a variable period but then begins to rise. Other features suggestive of myeloma or other diseases associated with monoclonal gammopathies are not initially present. Only a small fraction of individuals with **monoclonal gammopathies of undetermined significance (MGUS)** ultimately develop overt myeloma or another B-cell malignancy. Because of their age and the likelihood of other chronic disease processes, many die from intercurrent diseases before transformation to multiple myeloma can occur. Because we cannot predict accurately which patients will progress, however, all patients with MGUS require careful follow-up.

Primary Amyloidosis

Amyloidosis is a paraprotein disorder characterized by the extracellular deposition of a fibrillar protein with specific birefringent staining properties. When stained with Congo red and viewed with polarized light, it has an "apple-green" color. Because of its physical characteristics, particularly its insolubility and extensive extracellular deposition, it interferes with organ function. There are several types of amyloidosis, the most common of which is called **primary amyloidosis** or **AL amyloidosis**. This is a monoclonal disease characterized by tissue deposition of the variable portion of monoclonal immunoglobulin light chain, often in association with part or all of the constant region.

Amyloid fibrils consist of several individual protein filaments arranged in an antiparallel, beta-pleated sheet configuration, which confers the property of birefringence. Lambda light chains are more likely to form amyloid fibrils because of their physical and chemical properties. Nearly all patients with primary amyloidosis have either a monoclonal protein in the serum or a monoclonal light chain in the urine, but usually they do not show other features of myeloma such as an excess of plasma cells in the marrow.

Amyloid infiltration can occur in any organ; the major sites of deposition are the kidney, heart, gastrointestinal tract, liver, and autonomic nervous system. The kidney is the most common site of involvement, and the primary clinical manifestation is proteinuria, which occurs in 90% of patients. The proteinuria can progress to overt nephrotic syndrome (60%) and ultimately to renal failure and death (40% to 50%).

The heart is the most ominous site of involvement; cardiac involvement occurs in 60% of patients and usually results in death within 6 months. The major manifestations are refractory congestive heart failure, cardiac arrhythmia, and coronary artery disease caused by amyloid involvement of these vessels.

Involvement of the gastrointestinal tract can occur at any site. Manifestations include obstruction, bleeding, and malabsorption. One of the characteristic findings is macroglossia (enlargement of the tongue) caused by amyloid infiltration. Macroglossia occurs in 10% of patients with primary amyloid. When present, it constitutes an almost pathognomonic finding. Liver involvement is another common complication; amyloid infiltration can lead to massive hepatomegaly, often without marked impairment in hepatic function. Other sites of involvement include the autonomic nervous system, the carpal tunnel ligament, and the peripheral vasculature. Involvement of the peripheral vasculature can cause extreme muscle wasting. Primary amyloidosis can also lead to a bleeding diathesis as a result of absorption of clotting factor X by the abnormal protein.

Recent studies have shown that a diagnosis of amyloidosis can often be made by a simple aspirate of subcutaneous fat from the abdominal fat pad. When stained for amyloid, the aspirate can provide a diagnosis in over 80% of patients. Before the abdominal fat pad technique was developed, the most common means of diagnosis was rectal biopsy.

The amyloid associated with myeloma is identical to that oc-curring in primary amyloidosis, but other manifestations differ. The survival of patients with primary amyloidosis varies, averaging 17 months. Those with cardiac involvement have the shortest sur-vival, whereas those with only neurologic or carpal tunnel liga-ment involvement can survive for more than 5 years. Patients with amyloid associated with myeloma have a mean survival of only 4 months.

About 70% of amyloidosis of the AL type is a result of deposi-tion of the immunoglobulin light chains (primary amyloid and amyloid associated with myeloma). Morphologically identical ex-tracellular depositions of protein can occur as a secondary phenom-enon to several chronic diseases. This **secondary amyloidosis** is caused by the deposition of a portion of an acute phase reactant protein, serum amyloid A protein. The amyloid is termed **AA**. Amyloid A is not a paraprotein disease. There are several other forms of amyloid, including a number of inherited types. These also are not paraprotein disorders.

Lymphomas

Lymphomas are localized clonal neoplasms arising in areas of or-ganized lymphoid tissues. On the basis of the origin of the neoplas-tic cell, they are subdivided into two broad categories, **Hodgkin's disease (HD)** and **non-Hodgkin's lymphomas (NHLs)**.

Hodgkin's Disease

HD is a distinct neoplasm. The malignant cell in this tumor is the **Reed-Sternberg cell**, a large, multinucleated cell that may be derived from either lymphoid or monocytic precursors. Pathologi-cally, these cells are surrounded by numerous normal inflamma-tory cells, including lymphocytes, especially T cells; monocytes; and/or eosinophils. These inflammatory cells are believed to repre-sent the host defense response to either the tumor cells themselves or the inciting agent (e.g., an unknown virus). The greater the number of lymphocytes, the better the prognosis. Through immu-nophenotyping, most cells have been found to be T cells. If the T-cell response is inadequate, other cells, including B lymphocytes, macrophages, eosinophils, and plasma cells, form the infiltrate. Be-cause these cells are less able to control the proliferation of neoplas-tic cells, the disorder is more aggressive. HD is potentially curable.

Up to 80% of patients can be successfully treated with either chemotherapy or radiation.

Non-Hodgkin's Lymphomas

NHLs are malignancies of lymphocytes. In parallel with the normal division of lymphoid cells, NHLs can be caused by the neoplastic transformation of either T- or B-cell lymphocytes, but nearly all these malignancies are of B-cell origin. B-cell NHLs make up a heterogeneous group of neoplasms, ranging from low-grade diseases compatible with a long survival to high-grade tumors that, if untreated, are quickly fatal. These lymphomas are usually classified using categories agreed on by hematologists and hematopathologists, in classification schemes that are periodically updated.

The aggressiveness of a lymphoma can often be related to the specific stage of arrest in the normal B-cell maturation sequence. This concept has been incorporated into most systems used to classify and stage NHLs. Until very recently, the most widely used system for the classification of NHLs has been the Working Formulation, shown in Table 6–4. The Revised European American Lymphoma (REAL) classification (Table 6–5) was recently introduced. This classification is based on the presumed normal lymphoid counterparts and closely parallels the schemes used by hematopathologists in regular practice.

Low-grade diseases appear to represent the neoplastic transformation of cells arrested at the small B-lymphocyte stage. Like their normal counterparts, these tumor cells have a slow rate of replication. They also share another characteristic of normal lymphocytes, the ability to recirculate. Because of this migratory activity, the low-grade lymphomas are generally widely disseminated at the time of presentation.

In contrast, the more malignant variants, the intermediate- and high-grade lymphomas, simulate the morphologic and kinetic activities of antigen-stimulated normal lymphocytes. This stimulus induces the transformation of small, resting B lymphocytes into large, actively proliferating cells. High-grade lymphomas have a rapid turnover rate. Because these cells cannot recirculate, tumors may be localized at the time of presentation. Dissemination of these malignancies occurs by mechanisms similar to the spread of non-hematopoietic malignancies: direct extension and lymphatic and hematogenous routes.

Table 6–4 • Working Formulation: Classification of Non-Hodgkin's Lymphoma

1. Low-grade
   A. Malignant lymphoma, small lymphocytic
      (1) Chronic lymphocytic leukemia (CLL)
      (2) Plasmacytoid
   B. Malignant lymphoma, follicular, small cleaved cells
   C. Malignant lymphoma, follicular, mixed small cleaved and large cells
2. Intermediate-grade
   A. Malignant lymphoma, follicular, predominantly large cell
   B. Malignant lymphoma, diffuse, small cleaved cell
   C. Malignant lymphoma, diffuse, mixed small and large cell
   D. Malignant lymphoma, diffuse, large cell.
      (1) Cleaved cell
      (2) Noncleaved cell
3. High-grade
   A. Malignant lymphoma, large cell, immunoblastic
   B. Malignant lymphoma, lymphoblastic
   C. Malignant lymphoma, small noncleaved cell (Burkitt's)
4. Miscellaneous
   A. Composite
   B. Cutaneous T-cell lymphoma (mycosis fungoides, Sezary syndrome)
   C. "Histocytic"
   D. Extramedullary plasmacytoma
   E. Unclassified

As the name implies, the intermediate grades of NHL have clinical characteristics that are intermediate between the low- and high-grade lymphomas.

NHL has a predilection to occur in patients with immune deficiencies. For example, they are much more frequent in patients with congenital immune deficiencies such as Wiskott-Aldrich syndrome (thrombocytopenia, eczema, and recurrent infections); ataxia telangectasia (ataxia, telangiectasia, and recurrent sinopulmonary infections); and common variable hypogammaglobulinemia. Lymphomas are also common in HIV-infected patients and in those who have received either a solid organ or bone marrow transplant (post-transplant lymphoproliferative disease [PTLD]). In these latter groups, there is an association between infection with the Epstein-Barr virus and the lymphoma. The virus appears

Table 6–5 • Revised European-American Lymphoma Classification (REAL)

Precursor B-lymphoblastic lymphoma/leukemia
B-cell chronic lymphocytic leukemia/prolymphocytic leukemia/small lymphocytic lymphoma
Lymphoplasmacytoid lymphoma
Mantle-cell lymphoma

Follicular center lymphoma, follicular
• Grade I
• Grade II
• Grade III
Follicular center lymphoma, diffuse, small-cell (provisional)
Extranodal marginal zone B-cell lymphoma (low-grade B-cell lymphoma of MALT type)
Nodal marginal zone B-cell lymphoma (provisional)

Splenic marginal zone B-cell lymphoma (provisional)
Hairy-cell leukemia
Plasmacytoma/myeloma
Diffuse large B-cell lymphoma

Primary mediastinal large B-cell lymphoma
Burkitt's lymphoma
High-grade B-cell lymphoma, Burkitt-like (provisional)

Precursor T-lymphoblastic lymphoma/leukemia
T-cell chronic lymphocytic leukemia/prolymphocytic leukemia
Large granular lymphocytic leukemia
• T-cell type
• NK-cell type
Mycosis fungoides/Sezary syndrome

Peripheral T-cell lymphomas, unspecified (including provisional subtype: subcutaneous panniculitic T-cell lymphoma)

Hepatosplenic γ-δ T-cell lymphoma (provisional)
Angioimmunoblastic T-cell lymphoma

Source: Harris NL, Jaffe ES, Stein H, et al (1994). A revised European-American classification of lymphoid neoplasms: A proposal from the International Lymphoma Study Group. Blood 84:1361–1392, with permission.

to induce unregulated proliferation of B lymphocytes that are normally controlled by immunologically competent T cells. The malignancy actually arises as a result of a second inducing event, often the translocation of the *c-myc* gene (see the next-to-last paragraph on this page). In some transplant recipients, restoring immune competency by stopping immunosuppressive therapy causes spontaneous tumor regression.

The lymphomas arising in immunosuppressed patients share several common characteristics. They tend to be high-grade tumors that are often widely disseminated at presentation, occurring in extranodal sites, especially the gastrointestinal tract and the bone marrow. Central nervous system involvement is also common. These patients usually manifest "B"-type symptoms (unexplained fevers, night sweats, and weight loss). Response to therapy often produces a short period of remission, but overall survival is usually brief.

Another feature related to the pathogenesis of NHL is the association of specific tumors with chromosome abnormalities. Follicular-type lymphomas are associated with a translocation involving the 14 and 18 chromosomes t(14;18). This translocation brings the gene for the heavy chain of the immunoglobulin molecule on chromosome 14 in proximity to a gene termed *bcl-2* (B-cell lymphoma-2) on chromosome 18. The *bcl-2* gene controls apoptotic death of lymphocytes, and this translocation causes the elaboration of a protein that inhibits apoptosis, thus permitting prolonged survival of the neoplastic cells.

A second type of genetic abnormality occurs in the high-grade Burkitt's lymphoma: a translocation between chromosome 8 and one of the genes coding for portions of the immunoglobulin molecule. Most cases involve the heavy chain genes on chromosome 14, t(8;14). A few, however, show translocations with chromosomes 2, t(2;8) or 22, t(8;22), the two genes controlling light-chain synthesis. The locus for the kappa gene is on chromosome 2, and that for the lambda gene, on 22. All three types of translocations result in the juxtaposition of an oncogene, *c myc* on chromosome 8, to one of the genes responsible for immunoglobulin synthesis. It is believed that these abnormalities result in the unregulated and rapid growth of the lymphoma cells.

Clinical Manifestations of Lymphoma

The presenting manifestation of both Hodgkin's disease and non-Hodgkin's lymphoma is usually painless enlargement of one or more lymph nodes. As the disease progresses, nonlymphoid organs, such as the lungs, liver, or bone marrow, may be infiltrated with neoplastic lymphocytes. When the marrow is extensively involved, normal hematopoiesis can be suppressed, resulting in a pancytopenia. Both Hodgkin's and non-Hodgkin's lymphomas can produce systemic manifestations including fever, night sweats, and weight loss ("B" symptoms).

Although they have many clinical features in common, there are important differences between Hodgkin's disease and non-Hodgkin's lymphoma. The most important is malignant cell type. In Hodgkin's disease it is the Reed-Sternberg cell, whereas in NHL it is a neoplastic lymphocyte. The infiltrating lymphocytes in Hodgkin's disease are reactive cells. Hodgkin's disease has a unifocal origin (that is, it arises in one lymphoid area) and spreads contiguously. In non-Hodgkin's lymphomas, especially when low-grade, multifocal sites are common but the molecular changes are the same at all sites, indicating a unifocal origin as well. Thus HD usually spreads by continuity (adjacent lymph nodes are involved before distal nodes), whereas some NHLs appear to have noncontiguous dissemination (involvement of noncontiguous areas, such as the cervical and mesenteric lymph nodes, without involvement of other nodal areas).

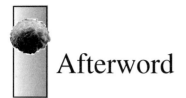

Afterword

This fifth edition of the *White Cell Manual* has featured leukocytes, one of the three major types of the formed elements of the blood. We have shown that leukocytes develop from pluripotent stem cells in the bone marrow and then enter the circulation and exert their critical host defense functions. These functions include phagocytic killing in the case of neutrophils and monocytes, antigen presentation in the case of HLA-DR positive monocytes and B lymphocytes, and cytokine expression in the case of monocytes and T lymphocytes. Cytokines facilitate other cellular activities. We have discussed the immunoglobulin-producing role of B lymphocytes and their derivative cells, the plasma cells, and seen the unfortunate effects of neoplastic proliferations of these cells. In considering the neoplastic proliferations of white blood cells, we have seen that these accumulations disrupt normal processes. Not only do neoplastic cells replace normal cells and deprive the host of their normal functions, they also affect immune functions. For instance, in chronic lymphocytic leukemia, in which nearly all of the B cells belong to a single antibody-forming clone, if these cells happened to produce antibody against a rare fruit fly, we would have plenty of this antibody but might have insufficient antibody against bacterial invaders.

Understanding how these cells may act in the larger scheme becomes clearer when we consider what could happen when a bacterial predator is introduced. Staphylococci are bacteria in our environment. We live in close contact with them, usually on peaceful terms. But under certain conditions, these bacteria gain the upper hand, leading to infirmities ranging from a pimple to lethal toxic shock syndrome. The cells discussed in this book act in concert to protect us from staphylococcal invasion. The "fable" below is adapted from well-known traditional verses to help you remember how it all works:

There is a place where staph hide.
You may get sick if you visit the place where staph hide.
But the staph are eaten by neutrophils, so you won't get sick if you visit the place where staph hide.

Antibodies coat the staph that are eaten by neutrophils so you won't get sick if you visit the place where staph hide.

B cells make the antibodies that coat the staph that are eaten by neutrophils so you won't get sick if you visit the place where staph hide.

Cytokines help the B cells make the antibodies that coat the staph that are eaten by neutrophils so you won't get sick if you visit the place where staph hide.

T cells make the cytokines that help the B cells make the antibodies that coat the staph that are eaten by neutrophils so you won't get sick if you visit the place where staph hide.

And would the little phagocyte
Prefer to dine by candlelight?
Or eat them quickly since it's able
As we've shown in our fable?

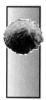

Bibliography

General References

Lee, G.R., Bithell, T.C., Foerster, J., Athens, J.W., & Lukens, J.N. (1993). Wintrobe's Clinical Hematology (9th edition). Philadelphia: Lea & Febiger.

Paul, W.E. (1993). Fundamental Immunology. New York: Raven Press.

Abbas, A.K., Lichtman, A.H., & Pober, J.S. (1994). Cellular & Molecular Immunology (2nd edition). Philadelphia: W. B. Saunders Co.

Stites, D.P., Terr, A.I., & Parslow, T.G. (1994). Basic & Clinical Immunology (8th edition). Norwalk, CT: Appleton & Lange.

Beutler, E., Lichtman, M.A., Coller, B.S., & Kipps, T. J. (1995). Williams' Hematology (5th edition). New York: McGraw-Hill Inc.

Hoffman, R., Benz, J.E.J., Shattil, S.J., Furie, B., Cohen, H.J., & Silberstein, L.E. (1995). Hematology, Basic Principles and Practice (2nd edition). New York: Churchill Livingstone.

Stem Cells

Cohen, J.J. (1985). Programmed cell death in the immune system. Adv. Immunol., 50, 55–89.

Schmitt, C., Eaves, C.J., & Lansdorp, P.M. (1991). Expression of CD34 on human B cell precursors. Clin. Exp. Immunol., 85, 168–173.

Civin, C., & Gore, S.D. (1993). Antigenic analysis of hematopoiesis: A review. J. Hematotherapy, 2, 137–144.

Ogawa, M. (1993). Differentiation and proliferation of hematopoietic stem cells. Blood, 81, 2844–2853.

Ogawa, M. (1994). Hematopoiesis. J. Allergy Clin. Immunol., 94, 645–650.

Growth Factors

Mosmann, T.R., & Coffman, R.L. (1985). Heterogeneity of cytokine secretion patterns and functions of helper T cells. Adv. Immunol., 46, 111–148.

Clark, S.C., & Kamen, R. (1987). The human hematopoietic colony-stimulating factor. Science, 236, 1229–1237.

Dinarello, C.A., & Mier, J.W. (1987). Lymphokines. N. Engl. J. Med., 317, 940–945.

Rowe, J.M., & Rapoport, A.P. (1992). Hematopoietic growth factors: A review. J. Clin. Pharmacol., 32, 486–501.

Oncology, A.S.C. (1994). Recommendations for the use of hematopoietic colony-stimulating factors: Evidence-based clinical practice guidelines. J. Clin. Oncol., 12, 2471–2508.

Sachs, L., & Lotem, J. (1994). The network of hematopoietic cytokines. Proc. Soc. Exp. Biol. Med., 206, 170–175.

Dale, D.C., Liles, W.C., Summer, W.R., & Nelson, S. (1995). Review: Granulocyte colony-stimulating factor—role and relationship to infectious disease. J. Infect. Dis., 173, 1061–1075.

McNiece, U.K., & Briddell, R.A. (1995). Stem cell factor. J. Leukoc. Biol., 58, 14–22.

Cohen, M.C., & Cohen, S. (1996). Cytokine function. Am. J. Clin. Pathol., 105, 589–598.

Fraser, J.K., Lill, M.C.C., & Figlin, R.A. (1996). The biology of the cytokine sequence cascade. Semin. Oncol., 23 (Suppl 4), 2–8.

Leukemias

General

Catovsky, D., & Matutes, E. (1992). The classification of acute leukemia. Leukemia, 6(Suppl 2), 1–6.

Ball, E.D. (1994). Leukemia. In J.M. Kirkwood, M.T. Lotze, & J.M. Yasko (Eds.), Current Cancer Therapeutics. Philadelphia: Princeton Academic Press, 186–192.

Sachs, L. (1996). The control of hematopoiesis and leukemia: From basic biology to the clinic. Proc. Natl. Acad. Sci. U.S.A., 93, 4742–4949.

Acute Myeloid Leukemia

Alcalay, M., Zangrilli, D., Pandolfi, P.P., et al (1991). Translocation breakpoint of acute promyelocytic leukemia lies within the retinoic acid receptors alpha locus. Proc. Natl. Acad. Sci. U.S.A., 88, 1977–1981.

Estey, E.H. (1995). Treatment of acute myelogenous leukemia and myelodysplastic syndromes. Semin. Hematol., 32, 132–151.

Lemons, R.S., Keller, S, Girtzen, D., et al. (1995). Acute promyelocytic leukemia. J. Pediatr. Hematol. Oncol., 17, 198–210.

Aplastic Anemia

Nissen, C. (1991). The pathophysiology of aplastic anemia. Semin. Hematol., 28, 313–318.

Young, N.S. (1995). Aplastic anemia. Lancet, 346, 228–232.

Chronic Myeloproliferative Disorders

Desforges, J.F., & Miller, K.B (1986). Blast crisis—reversing the direction. N. Engl. J. Med., 315, 1478–1479.

Kartarjian, H.M., Deisseroth, A., Kurzrock, R., et al. (1993). Chronic myelogenous leukemia: A concise update. Blood, 82, 691–703.

Myelodysplastic Syndromes

List, A.F., & Jacobs, A. (1992). Biology and pathogenesis of the myelodysplastic syndromes. Semin. Oncol., 19, 14–24.

Estey, E.H. (1995). Treatment of acute myelogenous leukemia and myelodysplastic syndromes. Semin. Hematol., 32, 132–151.

Hofmann, W.K., Ottmann, O.G., Ganser, A., & Hoelzer, D. (1996). Myelodysplastic syndromes: Clinical features. Semin. Hematol., 33, 177–185.

Bone Marrow Transplant

General

Armitage, J.O. (1994). Bone marrow transplantation. N. Engl. J. Med., 330, 827–838.

Storb, R. (1995). Bone marrow transplantation. Transplant Proc., 27, 2649–2652.

Walter, E.A., & Bowden, R.A. (1995). Infection in the bone marrow transplant recipient. Infect. Dis. Clin. North Am., 9, 823.

Antman, K. (1996). When are bone marrow transplants considered? Sci. Am., 275, 124–125.

Roman-Unfer, S., & Bitran, J.D. (1996). High-dose chemotherapy for malignancies: A review. Compr. Ther., 22, 107–120.

Russel, N., Gratwohl, A., & Schmitz, N. (1996). The place of blood stem cells in allogeneic transplantation. Br. J. Haematol., 93, 747–753.

Stem Cells

Morrison, S.J., Uchida, N., & Weissman, I.L. (1995). The biology of hematopoietic stem cells. Annu. Rev. Cell Biol. 11, 35–71.

Nash, R.A., & Storb, R. (1995). Transplantation of hematopoietic stem cells. Proc. Assoc. Am. Physicians, 107, 288–295.

Morrison, S.J., & Weissman, I.L. (1995). Heterogeneity of hematopoietic stem cells: Implications for clinical applications. Proc. Assoc. Am. Physicians, 107, 187–194.

Newburger, P.E., & Quesenberry, P.J., (1996). Umbilical cord blood as a new and promising source of unrelated-donor hematopoietic stem cells for transplantation. Curr. Opin. Pediatr., 8, 29–32.

Graft-Versus-Host Disease

Vandenberghe, P., & Boogaerts, M.A. (1995). Graft-versus-leukemia and graft-versus-lymphoma effects of allogeneic bone marrow transplantation and of allogeneic donor leukocyte transfusions. Ann. Hematol., 71, 209–217.

Barrett, A.J., & Malkovska (1996). Graft-versus-leukaemia: Understanding and using the alloimune response to treat haematologic malignancies. Br. J. Haematol., 93, 754–761.

Champlin, R., Giralt, S., & Gajewski, J. (1996). T cells, graft-versus-host disease and graft-versus-leukemia: Innovative approaches for blood and marrow transplantation. Acta Haematol., 95, 157–163.

Neutrophils

Reviews

Kaplan, S.S. (1995). Phagocytes. In H.R.J. & R.L. Simmons (Eds.), Surgical Infectious Disease. Norwalk, CT: Appleton Lange, pp. 247–276.

Host Defenses

Bodey, G.P., Buckley, M., Sathe, Y.S., et al. (1966). Quantitative relationship between circulating leukocytes and infections in patients with acute leukemia. Ann. Intern. Med., 64, 328–340.

Holmes, B., Qure, P.G., Windhorst, D.B., & Good, R.A. (1966). Fatal granulomatous disease of childhood. An inborn abnormality of phagocytic function. Lancet, 1(449), 1225–1228.

Malech, H.L., & Gallin, J.J. (1987). Neutrophils in human diseases. N. Engl. J. Med., 317, 687–694.

Lehrer, R.I., Ganz, T., Selsted, M.E., et al. (1988). Neutrophils and host defenses. Ann. Intern. Med. 109, 127–142.

Yang, K.D., & Hill, H.R. (1991). Neutrophil function disorders: Pathophysiology, prevention, and therapy. J. Pediatr., 119, 343–354.

Bogomolski-Yahalom, V., & Matzner, Y. (1995). Disorders of neutrophil functions. Blood Review, 9, 183–190.

Kinetics

Boggs, D.R. (1967). The kinetics of neutrophil leukocytes and in health and in disease. Semin. Hematol., 4, 359–417.

Adhesion

Zimmerman, G.A., Prescott, S.M., & McIntyre, T.M. (1992). Endothelial cell interaction with granulocytes: Tethering and signaling molecules. Immunol. Today, 13, 93–99.

Sharar, S.R., Winn, R.K., & Harlan, J.M. (1995). The adhesion cascade and anti-adhesion therapy: An overview. Springer Semin. Immunopathol., 16, 359–378.

Frenette, P.S., & Wagner, D.D. (1996). Adhesion molecules—Part I. N. Engl. J. Med., 334:1526–1529; and Part II: N. Engl. J. Med., 335, 43–45.

Eosinophils and Basophils

Silberstein, D.S. (1995). Eosinophil function in health and disease. Crit. Rev. Oncol. Hematol., 19, 47–77.

Thomas, L.L. (1995). Basophil and eosinophil interactions in health and disease. Chem. Immunol., 61, 186–207.

Wardlaw, A.J., Mogbel, R., & Kay, A.B. (1995). Eosinophils: Biology and role in disease. Adv. Immunol., 60, 151–266.

Martin, L.B., Kita, H., Leiferman, K.M, & Gleich, G.J. (1996). Eosinophils in allergy: role in disease, degranulation and cytokines. Internat. Arch. Allergy Immunol., 109, 207–215.

NADPH Oxidase

Sumimoto, H., Kenichiro, H., Kazuhito, M., et al. (1996). Assembly and activation of the phagocyte NADPH oxidase. J. Biol. Chem., 271, 22152–22158.

Wientjes, F.B., Panayotou, G., Reeves, E., & Segal, A.W. (1996). Interactions between cytosolic components of the NADPH oxidase: $p40^{phox}$ interacts with both $p67^{phox}$ and $p47^{phox}$. Biochem. J., 317, 919–924.

Monocytes

Whitelaw, D.M. (1972). Observations on human monocyte kinetics after pulse labeling. Cell Tissue Kinetics, 5, 311–317.

Unanue, E.R. (1978). The regulation of lymphocyte function by macrophages. Immunol. Rev., 40, 227.

Douglas, S.D., & Musson, R.A. (1986). Phagocytic defects—monocytes/macrophages. Clin. Immunol. Immunopathol., 40, 62.

Gordon, S. (1986). The biology of the macrophage. J. Cell Sci. (Suppl), 4, 267.

Johnston, R.B.J. (1986). Monocytes and macrophages. N. Engl. J. Med., 318, 574.

Nathan, C.F. (1987). Secretory products of macrophages. J. Clin. Invest., 79, 319–326.

Unanue, E. R., & Allan, P.M. (1987). The basis for the immunoregulatory role of macrophages and other accessory cells. Science, 236, 51–57.

Stein, M., & Keshav, S. (1993). The versatility of macrophages. Clin. Exp. Allergy, 22, 19–27.

Tapper, H. (1996). The secretion of preformed granules by macrophages and neutrophils. J. Leuk. Biol., 59, 613–622.

Lymphocytes

Cohen, J.J. (1985). Programmed cell death in the immune system. Adv. Immunol., 50, 55–86.

Fowlkes, B.J., & Pardoll, D.M. (1989). Molecular and cellular events of T cell development. Int. Archives of Allergy and Immunology, 105, 203–210.

Parnes, J.R. (1989). Molecular biology and function of CD4 and CD8. Adv. Immunol., 44, 265–312.

Banchereau, J., & Rousset, F. (1992). Human lymphocytes: Phenotype, proliferation and differentiation. Adv. Immunol., 52, 125–262.

Paulnock, D.M. (1992). Macrophage activation by T cells. Curr. Opin. Immunol., 4, 344–349.

Rothenberg, E.V. (1992). The development of human T and natural killer cells. Adv. Immunol., 51, 85–214.

Lanier, L.L. (1993). Distribution and function of lymphocyte surface antigens. Ann. N.Y. Acad. Sci., 677, 86–93.

Stoolman, L.M. (1993). Adhesion molecules involved in leukocyte recruitment and lymphocyte recirculation. Chest, 103 (suppl), 79S–86S.

van Noesel, C.J.M., & van Lierm, R.A.W. (1993). Architecture of the human B-cell antigen receptor. Blood 82, 363–373.

He, W., and Kabelitz, D. (1994). Cytokines involved in intrathymic T cell development. Int. Arch. Allergy Immunol. 105, 203–210.

Picker, L.J. (1994). Control of lymphocyte homing. Curr. Opin. Immunol., 6, 394–406.

Billips, L.G., Lassoued, K., Nunez, C., et al. (1995). Human B-cell development. Ann. N.Y. Acad. Sci., 764, 1–8.

Spits, H.L., & Phillips, J.H. (1995). Development of human T and natural killer cells. Blood, 85, 2654–2670.

Springer, T.A. (1995). Traffic signals in endothelium for lymphocyte recirculation and leukocyte emigration. Ann. Rev. Physiol., 57, 827–872.

Immune Deficiencies

Hong, R. (1990). Update on the immunodeficiency diseases. Am. J. Dis. Child., 144, 983–992.

Preud'homme, J.L., & Hanson, L.A. (1990). IgG subclass deficiency. Immunodeficiency Review, 2, 129–149.

Buckley, R.H. (1992). Immunodeficiency disease. JAMA, 268, 2797–2806.

Rosen, F.S. (Chairman) (1992). Primary immunodeficiency diseases. Report of a WHO scientific group. Immunodeficiency Reviews, 3, 195–236.

Gaidano, G., Pastore, C., Lanza, C., & Mazza, U. (1994). Molecular pathology of AIDS-related lymphomas. Ann. Hematol., 69, 281–290.

Rosen, F.S., Cooper, M.D., & Wedgewood, R.J. (1995). The primary immunodeficiencies. N. Engl. J. Med., 333, 431–440.

B-Cell Malignancies

Foon, K.A., Rai, K.R., & Gale, R.P. (1990). Chronic lymphocytic leukemia: New insight into biology and therapy. Ann. Intern. Med., 113, 525–539.

Shirai, T., Hirose, S., Okada, T., & Nishimura, H. (1991). CD5+ B cells in autoimmune disease and lymphoid malignancy. Clin. Immunol. Immunpathol., 59, 173–186.

Barlogie, B., & Gale, R.P. (1992). Multiple myeloma and chronic lymphocytic leukemia: Parallels and contrasts. Am. J. Med., 93, 443–450.

Skinner, M. (1992). Protein AA/SAA. J. Intern. Med., 232, 513–514.

Freeman, A.S., & Nadler, L.M. (1993). Immunologic markers in B-cell chronic lymphocytic leukemia. In B.D. Cheson (Ed.), Chronic Lymphocytic Leukemia. New York: Marcel Dekker, pp. 1–32.

Mulligan, S.P., & Catovsky, D. (1993). The chronic B-cell leukaemias. Aust. N.Z. J. Med., 23, 42–50.

Youinou, P., Mackenzie, L., Lamour, A.J., et al. (1993). Human CD5+ B cells and autoimmunity. Ist. J. Med. Sci., 29, 151–153.

Alexanian, R., & Dimopoulous, M. (1994). The treatment of multiple myeloma. N. Engl. J. Med., 330, 484–489.

Harris, N.L., Jaffe, E.S., Stein, H., et al. (1994). A revised European-American classification of lymphoid neoplasms: A proposal from the International Study Group. Blood, 84, 1361–1392.

Aisenberg, A.C. (1995). Coherent view of non-Hodgkin's lymphoma. J. Clin. Oncol., 13:2656–2675.

Bakkus, M.H.C., van Riet, I., de Greef, C., et al. (1995). The clonogenic precursor cell in multiple myeloma. Leukemia Lymphoma, 18, 221–229.

Choukroun, G., Varet, B., & Grunfeld, J.P. (1995). Multiple myeloma, Part 1: Renal involvement. Nephron, 70, 11–17.

Klein, B., Zhang, X.G., Lu, Z.Y., & Bataille, R. (1995). Interleukin-6 in human multiple myeloma. Blood, 85, 863–873.

O'Brien, S., del Giglio, A., & Keating, M. (1995). Advances in the biology and treatment of B-cell chronic lymphocytic leukemia. Blood, 85, 307–318.

Rozman, C., & Montserrat, E. (1995). Chronic lymphocytic leukemia. N. Engl. J. Med., 333, 1052–1057.

Vartersian, M.L. (1995). Biologic and clinical advances in multiple myeloma. Oncology 9, 417–424.

Freedman, A.S. (1996). Cell surface antigens in leukemias and lymphomas. Cancer Invest., 14, 252–276.

Kwak, L.W., & Longo, D.L.: Lymphomas (1996). Cancer Chemother. Biol. Response Modif., 16, 376.

Schiffer, M. (1996). Molecular anatomy and pathological expression of antibody light chains. Am. J. Pathol., 148, 1339–1344.

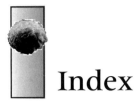

Index